Shoulder Injuries and Treatment

Edited by Nahum Rosenberg

Published in London, United Kingdom

Shoulder Injuries and Treatment
http://dx.doi.org/10.5772/intechopen.1008021
Edited by Nahum Rosenberg

Contributors
Adeera Azam, Alberto Roldán-Ruiz, Andrew Ames, Benjamin Sanderford, Elżbieta Sawicka-Garbarek, Emine Merve Ersever, Esha Dilawar, Gabriele Bertotti, Hubert Laprus, Il-Tae Jang, Ishal Ayub, Jiekai Ye, Joanna Walecka, Kelly Wolfe, Kiran Shahzadi, Kyun-Ho Shin, Lyba Musaddiq, Marta Jokiel, Muhammad Hafeez, Muhammad Suleman Tahir, Neal Krentz, Panpan Xie, Seung-Beom Han, Shabana Rahim, Shuhua Lan, Shuming Huang, Svetoslav Dobrilov

First published in London, United Kingdom, 2025 by IntechOpen
IntechOpen is the global imprint of INTECHOPEN LIMITED, registered in England and Wales, registration number: 11086078, 167-169 Great Portland Street, London, W1W 5PF, United Kingdom

For EU product safety concerns: IN TECH d.o.o., Prolaz Marije Krucifikse Kozulić 3, 51000 Rijeka, Croatia, info@intechopen.com or visit our website at intechopen.com.

British Library Cataloguing-in-Publication Data
A catalogue record for this book is available from the British Library

Shoulder Injuries and Treatment
Edited by Nahum Rosenberg
p. cm.
Print ISBN 978-1-83635-340-9
Online ISBN 978-1-83635-339-3
eBook (PDF) ISBN 978-1-83635-341-6

Meet the editor

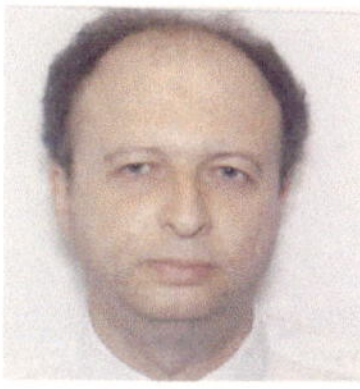

Nahum Rosenberg, MD, Ph.D., MOrthop, MBA, FRCS (England), is an orthopedic consultant surgeon with over 30 years of experience in the field. He graduated with an MD from the Faculty of Medicine, Technion Israel Institute of Technology in 1990 and obtained a Ph.D. from the University of Portsmouth, UK. He completed his orthopedic surgery residency at Rambam Medical Center in 1997 and earned an MOrthop degree from Tel Aviv University in 1996. Dr. Rosenberg served as a Nuffield Fellow at Oxford University (1998-1999) and completed clinical fellowships in Australia and at the University of Nottingham, UK. Since 2003, he has worked as a senior orthopedic surgeon at Rambam Health Care Campus and became an assistant clinical professor at Technion-IIT in 2007. He has authored 90 peer-reviewed articles, 5 books, and given 150 international presentations, while serving on the editorial boards of ten orthopedic journals.

Contents

Preface

The shoulder represents one of the most complex and fascinating joints in the human body, a remarkable structure that sacrifices inherent stability for extraordinary mobility. This unique biomechanical arrangement, while enabling the remarkable range of motion that defines human upper extremity function, also renders the shoulder particularly vulnerable to a diverse spectrum of injuries and pathological conditions.

Shoulder Injuries and Treatment emerges from the recognition that effective shoulder care requires a comprehensive, evidence-based approach that extends far beyond traditional boundaries. In an era where patients—from weekend warriors to elite athletes—demand not merely pain relief but complete restoration of function and return to active lifestyles, clinicians must be equipped with both foundational knowledge and innovative treatment strategies.

This volume addresses the full continuum of shoulder pathology, from acute traumatic injuries such as anterior dislocations and glenoid fractures to complex chronic conditions, including multidirectional instability and massive rotator cuff tears. What distinguishes this text is its commitment to presenting both surgical and non-surgical interventions within a framework that recognizes the profound interconnections between structure, function, and the broader biopsychosocial context of healing.

The chapters within reflect a paradigm shift toward more holistic care. Rather than viewing the shoulder in isolation, contributors explore the cervical spine's often-overlooked contribution to shoulder pain, emphasize the critical role of manual therapy as a cornerstone of conservative treatment, and advocate for rehabilitation approaches that address not only biomechanical deficits but also neuromuscular control and psychological factors that influence recovery.

For the surgical patient, this book presents both established procedures and innovative techniques. From the evolving landscape of total shoulder arthroplasty in active athletes to cost-effective approaches, such as superior capsular reconstruction using autologous biceps tendon, the surgical content reflects current best practices while acknowledging the paramount importance of appropriate patient selection and comprehensive rehabilitation.

The emphasis throughout is on evidence-based practice, individualized care, and optimization of functional outcomes. Each chapter provides clinicians with the tools necessary to develop treatment algorithms that can be tailored to the unique needs, goals, and circumstances of each patient.

This book serves as an essential resource for orthopedic surgeons, sports medicine physicians, physical therapists, and all healthcare providers involved in the care of the shoulder. Students and residents will find comprehensive foundational knowledge, while experienced practitioners will appreciate the integration of cutting-edge research with practical clinical applications.

As we continue to refine our understanding of shoulder biomechanics and expand our therapeutic arsenal, the principles outlined in this volume—comprehensive assessment, evidence-based treatment selection, and holistic rehabilitation—will remain the cornerstones of excellent shoulder care. We hope that this resource will contribute to improved outcomes and an enhanced quality of life for the countless patients who entrust us with their care.

The journey toward optimal shoulder health is rarely straightforward. Still, with the knowledge, techniques, and perspectives presented in these pages, clinicians are better equipped to guide their patients successfully along that path.

Nahum Rosenebrg
National Insurance Institute,
Haifa, Israel

Section 1

Foundational Concepts and Assessment

Chapter 1

Shoulder Rehabilitation

Adeera Azam, Ishal Ayub, Lyba Musaddiq, Esha Dilawar and Muhammad Suleman Tahir

Abstract

Shoulder joint is a complex and highly mobile joint as it is a less stable and highly mobile joint in human body. Due to less stability, it is more prone to injuries and joint dysfunction. This chapter provides evidence-based comprehensive overview about restoring shoulder function and range following injury, chronic musculoskeletal conditions, and surgery. It starts with the detailed explanation of anatomy and biomechanics of shoulder joint, emphasizing the balance between stability and mobility of joint surrounded by different static and dynamic structures. This chapter explores common shoulder pathologies, that is, adhesive capsulitis, rotator cuff tear, shoulder impingement syndrome and dislocations. This chapter also emphasizes the importance of shoulder rehabilitation strategies including electrotherapeutic modalities, shoulder mobilizations, and active and passive exercises. This chapter also outlines different assessment techniques to rule out/differentiate different dysfunctions. Special attention is given to pain management, neuromuscular and proprioceptive control, and improvement in ROM and return to function protocols. This chapter provides a complete evidence-based guide for clinicians, therapists, and students involved in the rehabilitation of various shoulder disorders.

Keywords: shoulder joint, adhesive capsulitis, rotator cuff tear, shoulder rehabilitation, shoulder mobilization, pain management

1. Introduction

Most shoulder injuries occur due to micro-trauma or macro-trauma, whether it is caused by overhead shoulder activities or enough force applied to the shoulder joint. Overhead movement causes abnormal stresses on joints and makes them more vulnerable to injuries or dislocations. Shoulder injuries are also common in players as well due to overuse or altered biomechanics of the shoulder joint. Conte et al. reported that 28% of all injuries present among baseball pitchers were related to the shoulder joint. This chapter reviews the anatomical structures enabling these different types of movements and examines the biomechanics and different rehabilitation approaches.

1.1 Structure of the shoulder

1.1.1 Anatomy and biomechanics

The shoulder joint is known as the shoulder complex. The glenohumeral joint, sternoclavicular joint, acromioclavicular joint, coracoclavicular joint, and scapulothoracic joints are the five distinct articulations, along with ligaments, bursas, and rotator cuff muscles, that make up the shoulder, the most complicated and complex joint in the human body. Sternoclavicular, acromioclavicular, and glenohumeral components are true joints. Dysfunction in any of these structures limits the performance of the shoulder complex [1].

1.1.2 Sternoclavicular joint (SC)

The sternoclavicular joint is where the end of the collarbone meets the cartilage of the first rib and the notch on the top part of the breastbone. It is a modified saddle joint, which connects the shoulder complex with the thorax. The costoclavicular ligament acts as a primary stabilizer for this joint. This ligament checks the elevation of the clavicle and stabilizes the joint anteriorly and posteriorly [2]. The SC joint allows free motion in the frontal and transverse planes as well as some rotations in the forward and backward sagittal planes. A fibrocartilaginous articular disc functions as a shock absorber and enhances the fit of the articulating bone surfaces. When performing movements like swimming, raising the arms above the head, and shrugging the shoulders, rotation takes place at the SC joint. The close-packed position for the SC joint is maximal shoulder elevation [2, 3].

1.1.3 Acromioclavicular joint

The acromioclavicular joint is an irregular plane joint between acromion process of the scapula and the distal end of clavicle. Despite having restricted motion in all three planes due to its construction, it is classified as an irregular diarthrodial joint. AC joint has two primary functions: (1) During early stage of upper limb elevation, it maintains relationship between scapula and clavicle and (2) in later stage of upper limb elevation provides additional range of rotation to thorax [1]. The coracoclavicular ligament acts as a primary stabilizer of AC joint. This ligament is responsible for controlling the linear rotation of clavicle which is crucial for fully unrestricted upper limb elevation. Anteroposterior stability of joint is maintained by joint capsule and longitudinal stability is maintained by coracoclavicular ligament. When the humerus is abducted to 90°, the AC joint is in its close-packed position [2].

1.1.4 Coracoclavicular joint

The syndesmosis between the inferior surface of the clavicle and the coracoid process of the scapula, joined by the coracoclavicular ligament, is known as the coracoclavicular joint. There is hardly much movement possible at this joint [3].

1.1.5 Glenohumeral joint

It is a synovial joint of the ball and socket variety formed between the glenoid cavity of the scapula and the head of the humerus. It is the most mobile and least stable

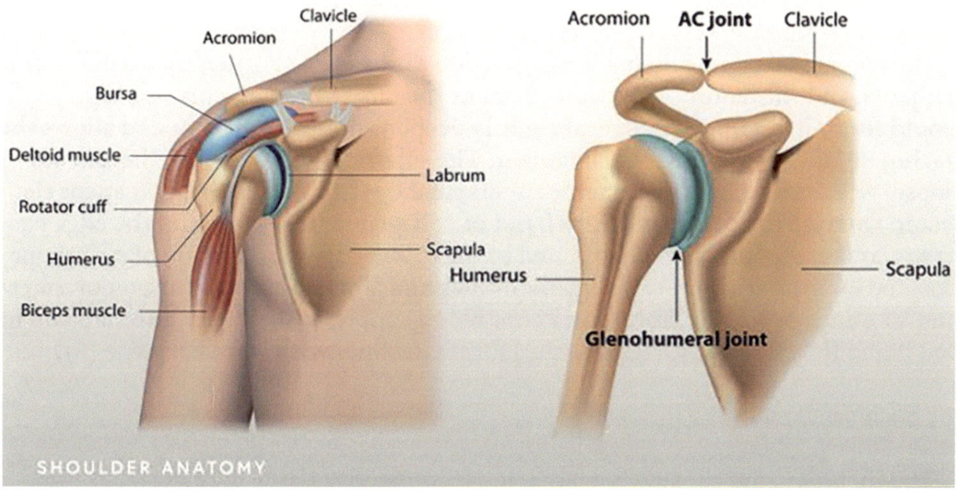

Figure 1.
Anatomy of shoulder joint [4].

joint in the human body, which enables the movement of the shoulder in all planes. It is an inherently unstable joint due to its bony articulation. Compared to the shallow glenoid fossa of the scapula with which it articulates, the nearly hemispherical head of the humerus has three to four times the surface area. It is also the most commonly dislocated joint in the human body. At the extremes of the range of motion, there are significant translations of the humeral head on the glenoid fossa when the arm is passively rotated (**Figure 1**) [5].

The stabilization of humeral head within glenoid cavity is maintained by both static and dynamic stabilizers (**Table 1**) [3].

1.1.6 Shoulder stabilizers

Each person has a different anatomical shape for the glenoid fossa; around 45% of people have an oval shape, while the remaining 55% have a pear-shaped cavity. The inferior half of the glenoid cavity is 20% larger than the superior half, and the articulating area of the glenoid fossa is much smaller than the humeral head. During normal movement of the arm, only 25 to 30% of the humeral head comes in contact with the glenoid cavity. This lack of articular contact leads to instability of the joint. The glenoid faces superiorly, laterally, and anteriorly, which limits inferior translation of the humeral head on the glenoid. Bony defects in either the humeral head or glenoid are associated with shoulder instability and recurrent dislocations [5].

Static	Dynamic
Bone geometry, glenohumeral ligaments, glenoid labrum, and capsule	Predominantly rotator cuff muscles
	Scapular stabilizers
	Trapezius, levator scapulae, serratus anterior, rhomboids

Table 1.
Shoulder static and dynamic stabilizers [3].

1.1.7 The glenoid labrum

The glenoid labrum, a lip made of a portion of the joint capsule, the glenohumeral ligaments, and the tendon of the long head of the biceps brachii, surrounds the glenoid fossa. It is a fibrous rim that slightly deepens the glenoid fossa and allows the attachment of the glenohumeral ligament. The superior attachment of the labrum is loose, whereas the inferior attachment is somehow firm. The labrum deepens the glenoid from 2.5 to 5 mm. This thick band of collagenous tissue around the edge has a triangular cross section, which is joined to the fossa's edge. So, this rim of soft tissue is located on the periphery of the glenoid fossa and adds stability to the glenohumeral joint. The anterosuperior labrum has poor blood supply, while the inferior labrum has good blood flow. The vascularity of the labrum declines with increasing age [6].

1.1.8 Shoulder capsule and ligaments

The shoulder joint capsule is a large, loose connective tissue that allows a large degree of shoulder range of motion and contributes to joint stability. The glenohumeral joint capsule is supported by glenohumeral ligaments that add to joint stability. The anterior glenohumeral ligament prevents anterior translation of the humerus on the glenoid. The superior and middle glenohumeral ligaments also prevent anterior translation when the arm is 180 degrees abducted. The middle glenohumeral ligament plays an important role in limiting the humeral head on the glenoid when the shoulder is in the mid-range of abduction. The inferior glenohumeral ligament prevents translation when the arm is abducted at 90 degrees or beyond [7].

1.1.9 Dynamic stabilizers

The most important function of primary glenohumeral stabilizers is to provide combined muscular contraction that enhances humeral stability during active arm movements. These muscles work together in an agonist and antagonist fashion to provide the movement and stability at one point in time. The joint capsule is also joined by the tendons of four muscles. Due to their role in humeral rotation and the formation of a collagenous cuff around their tendons, these muscles are referred to as the rotator cuff muscles. These include supraspinatus, infraspinatus, teres minor, and subscapularis. They are also occasionally referred to as the SITS muscles, which is derived from the first letter of their names. The subscapularis aids in medial rotation, whereas the supraspinatus, infraspinatus, and teres minor aid in lateral rotation of GH joint [8].

The head of the humerus is pulled toward the glenoid fossa by tension in the rotator cuff muscles, which significantly reduces the joint's little stability. It has been demonstrated that the biceps and rotator cuff muscles are engaged to stabilize the shoulder before the humerus moves. Additionally, the glenohumeral joint is stabilized by the negative pressure inside its capsule. Humerus abduction and external rotation are closed pack position of shoulder joint. Neuromuscular control is also a component that adds stability in shoulder joint. This factor is most important to normal shoulder function than joint position or repositioning ability [9].

1.1.10 Scapulothoracic joint

The joint between the anterior scapula and the thoracic wall is frequently referred to as the scapulothoracic joint since the scapula can move in both the sagittal and frontal planes with regard to the spine. There are two purposes for the muscles that attach to the scapula. They might first contract to stabilize the area of the shoulder. For instance, when a suitcase is raised off the floor, tension is created in the levator scapula, trapezius, and rhomboids to support the scapula, and consequently, the entire shoulder *via* the acromioclavicular joint. Second, the muscles of the scapula can help to move the glenohumeral joint in the proper position to support the upper extremity [10].

1.1.11 Bursae

The shoulder region contains a number of tiny, fibrous sacs that release synovial fluid. These sacs, called bursae, act as a cushion and lessen friction between collagenous tissue layers. A number of bursae, including the subscapularis, subcoracoid, and subacromial, encircle the shoulder. The subscapularis and subcoracoid bursae are in charge of controlling the friction between the subscapularis muscle's superficial fibers and the humeral head, the coracoid process, and the scapular neck. The subacromial bursa is located in the subacromial space, which is situated between the glenohumeral joint (below) and the scapula's acromion process and coracoacromial ligament (above). The rotator cuff muscles, especially the supraspinatus, are cushioned by this bursa from the bone acromion above. Compressing the subacromial bursa repeatedly during overhead arm motion can irritate it (**Figure 2**) [12].

1.1.12 Scapulohumeral rhythm

A consistent scapular rotation pattern that supports and aids with humeral abduction. Two thirds of the motion when the arm is fully raised by abduction or flexion takes place at the glenohumeral joint, with the other third occurring between the scapula and thorax. Scapulohumeral rhythm is the term used to describe this coordinated movement. The glenohumeral supraspinatus typically initiates the initial few degrees of shoulder abduction during the first 30 degrees of abduction/flexion.

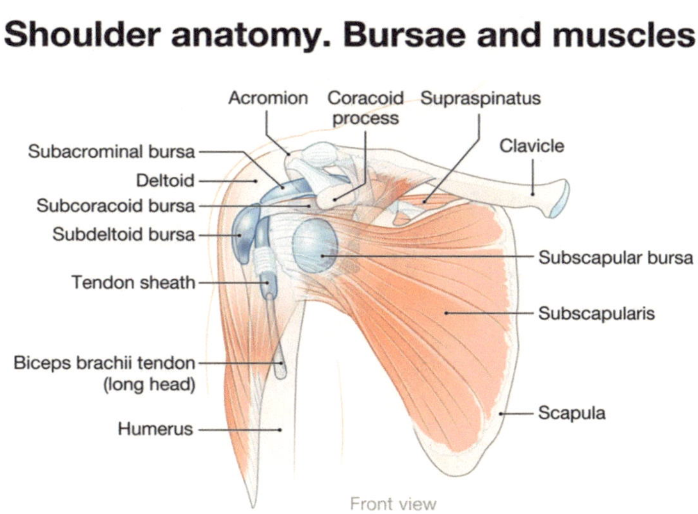

Figure 2.
Bursae of shoulder joint [11].

Scapulothoracic and glenohumeral joints move in tandem with the remaining elevation, with a 2:1 ratio of glenohumeral to scapulothoracic movement. Scapulohumeral rhythm prevents from shoulder impingement [13].

2. Types of shoulder injuries

2.1 Overuse injuries

Bursitis, tendinitis (rotator cuff, biceps tendon, or both), and degenerative or post-traumatic arthritis are examples of overuse injuries of the shoulder. The elements of overuse are repetitive activities and vigorous overhead movements, that is, swimming, throwing. Overuse injuries are also frequently caused by impingement syndrome, which is the impingement of the periarticular soft tissues between the coracoacromial arch and the larger tuberosity of the humerus [14].

There are several possible causes of impingement.

Glenohumeral instability can be post-traumatic, as is frequently observed following a shoulder injury, or atraumatic, as is frequently observed in swimmers and throwers. Narrowing of the subacromial space results from glenohumeral instability, which causes the humeral head to translate further in the anterosuperior direction. Weakness and inflammation are the results of the impingement on the rotator cuff tendons [15]. Additionally, excessive scapular protraction and rotation can lead to impingement and worse acromion mobility when the rotator cuff muscles and the scapular stabilizing muscles (rhomboids, trapezius, and levator scapulae) are not balanced. Impingement, instability, or both, in conjunction with an acute overuse syndrome, frequently result in the inflammatory condition that causes a patient's pain.

Complete rehabilitation depends on treating the acute inflammatory disease while paying close attention to the underlying fundamental problem [16].

2.2 Trauma

Contusions, fractures, dislocations, subluxations, separations, and traumatic impingement are the several categories of shoulder trauma. Usually, the clavicle, proximal humerus, or both are affected by fractures.

The majority of shoulder dislocations occur anteriorly (90%) and less frequently posteriorly (10%). Unfortunately, the rate of missed diagnoses for posterior shoulder dislocations is intolerable. Additionally, a shoulder subluxation is sometimes disregarded as the reason why patients experience pain or functional instability. One of the most frequent shoulder illnesses, acromioclavicular separation can range in severity. Last but not least, traumatic impingement frequently causes a partial or total rotator cuff tear, particularly in people over 40 [17].

3. Shoulder assessment

A comprehensive *history and physical examination* are the first steps in properly evaluating any shoulder problem. The most common presenting sign of shoulder injuries is pain and sometimes accompanied by weakness. Most of the time, a thorough history results in an accurate diagnosis. Finding the triggering event is crucial for both acute injuries and overuse injuries [12].

It is important to take into account the patient's age, occupation, side of dominance, history of prior shoulder illnesses, and shoulder position at the time of injury, the mechanism of injury and direction of force as well. Pain during overhead or throwing activities may be a sign of impingement, instability, or both in cases of overuse injuries. An inflammatory condition is represented by pain that is worse at night or after using the affected shoulder.

Patients with shoulder pain who do not have a history of trauma or overuse should have any major underlying causes, such as systemic arthritis, infection, cancer, or heart disease, ruled out [18].

It is essential to expose both shoulders sufficiently to identify any small asymmetry. The appearance of visible deformity brought on by fractures or dislocations, edema, erythema, ecchymosis, or muscular atrophy should receive special attention [19].

Range of motion (ROM) exercises that is active are subsequently carried out and contrasted with those in the shoulder that is asymptomatic. Active range of motion exercises should also be viewed from behind since shoulder movements require moving the scapula. A painful arc of motion, typically between 60 and 120 degrees of abduction, is the indicative of impingement syndrome in overuse injuries [20].

Weakness, pain, or both may be the cause of a restriction in an active range of motions. A total rotator cuff tear is indicated by an inability to abduct the arm. With or without a restriction in active range of motion, partial rotator cuff tears are frequently accompanied by pain or noticeable weakness on strength testing. Passive ROM can assist in identifying the cause of restricted active ROM. Passive range of motion should not be limited in cases of overuse injuries. Active and passive ROM restriction points to either adhesive capsulitis or a frozen shoulder. The most notable finding in this case is a restriction on external rotation [21].

Pain from traumatic sources can limit both active and passive ranges of motion, particularly when there is fracture or dislocation. Proximal humeral fractures and dislocations are challenging to diagnose, and it has been estimated that up to 80% of posterior locked dislocations go unnoticed by the first treating physician [22].

Certain tests, such the Jobe's and Speed's tests, are helpful in determining the integrity of the supraspinatus and biceps tendons, respectively. The location of the discomfort and dysfunction is then determined by palpation. In contrast to acute trauma injury, which causes more localized pain, overuse injuries frequently cause more widespread pain. It is easy to feel the biceps tendon in its groove directly medial to the larger tuberosity over the humeral head. Bicipital tendinitis is associated with palpable tenderness and pain on Speed's test (**Figures 3** and **4**) [25].

When a shoulder dislocation occurs, the humeral head can frequently be felt either anteriorly or posteriorly in relation to the glenoid, and upon examination, there is a noticeable visual abnormality. Several maneuvers can reveal glenohumeral instability. Attempts are made to slide the humeral head both anteriorly and posteriorly by supporting the scapula with one hand while palpating the humeral head through the deltoid [26].

Anterior instability can also be assessed using the apprehension test. The patient is seated, and the examiner rotates the abducted arm externally puts strain on the proximal humerus from the front. A "positive" result occurs when the patient feels as though a subluxation is about to happen or when their muscles are strained. When direct longitudinal pressure on the humerus causes a palpable deficiency beneath the acromion, known as the "sulcus" sign, inferior laxity may be apparent. With a history of the shoulder "popping out," nonspecific glenohumeral pain, and associated

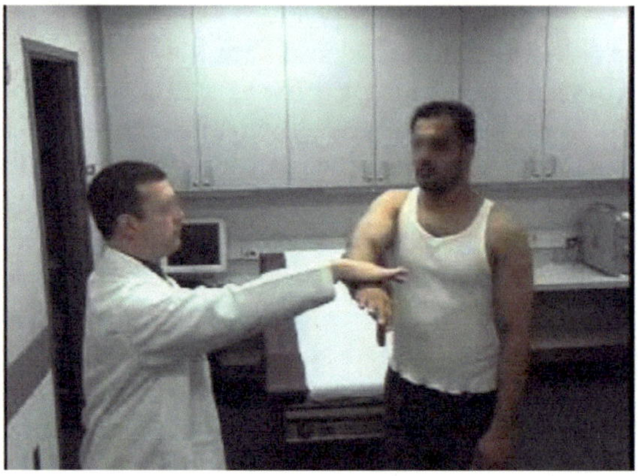

Figure 3.
Speed test [23].

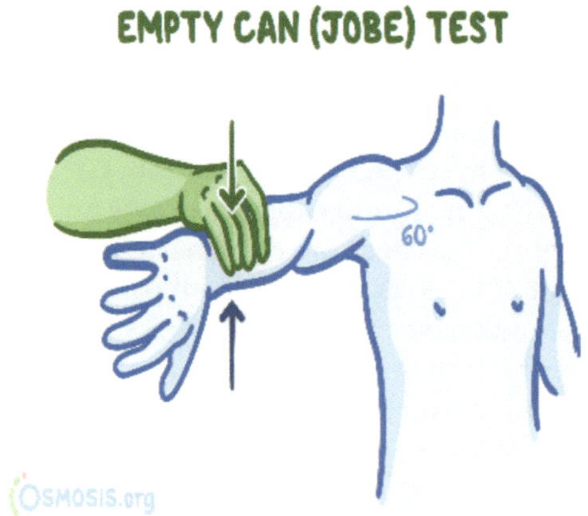

Figure 4.
Jobe's test [24].

symptoms including numbness, tingling, weakness, and bouts of a "dead arm," such an abnormal finding would support a diagnosis of shoulder subluxation [27].

Since there may be damage to the brachial or radial arteries (or both), as well as injury to the axillary, musculocutaneous, and ulnar nerves, associated neurovascular structures should always be assessed, particularly in traumatic shoulder conditions [28].

When diagnosing shoulder injuries, plain radiographs in both AP and lateral view are the initial imaging step. Both are crucial for accurately diagnosing dislocations and fractures.

About 75% of chronic dislocations and 25% of initial anterior dislocations will be accompanied by a compression fracture of the posterolateral portion of the humeral head. Further AP views with internal or external rotation are especially helpful in proximal humeral fractures and will show the lesser and greater tuberosities of the humeral head, respectively [29].

In addition to typical AP and axillary views, a genuine AP view (40 degrees postero-oblique projection) will display the glenoid in perspective to evaluate for overuse problems. Acromial anatomy is a crucial finding in patients who may have suspected impingement because this syndrome may be exacerbated by a curved or hooked acromion. Calcium deposits might indicate bursitis or calcific tendinitis. Degenerative alterations surrounding the glenoid, such as sclerosis, osteophytic lipping, or both, indicate instability or previous subluxation or dislocation [30].

Other diagnostic procedures include magnetic resonance imaging, computed tomography (CT), and CT arthrography. In some circumstances, fluoroscopy or magnetic resonance imaging (MRI) may be recommended. The preferred diagnostic method for demonstrating soft tissue features like the rotator cuff or labral ligaments is magnetic resonance imaging with contrast. For trauma or to further define bone pathology, computed tomographic scanning is helpful. In situations when MRI scanning is not feasible, computed tomographic arthrography can be helpful. When available, magnetic resonance imaging (MRI) is replacing fluoroscopy as the method of diagnosis for impingement [31].

4. Shoulder injuries and joint pathologies

4.1 Rotator cuff tears

Four muscles make up the rotator cuff, which are supraspinatus, infraspinatus, subscapularis, and teres minor. They attach to the humeral head *via* tendons and are the key components that maintain shoulder function and stability. Any tear or detachment of a tendon joining these muscles to humerus is known as a rotator cuff tear [32].

Since Codman in the 1930s, many theories have been proposed to explain the origin of rotator cuff tears. Here, we go into the supporting evidence that these concepts, which generally fall into "intrinsic" and "extrinsic" arguments. Neer originally put forward the impingement theory, the most renowned extrinsic pathogenic component of cuff illness. According to Neer, acromial morphology was essential for the process of partial tears, which eventually culminated in full-thickness tears due to repetitive movement of the cuff beneath the acromion. Bigliani et al. categorized acromions into three pathogenic groups: Type I, or flat, makes up 17% of cuff tears, and Type II, or curved, and Type III, or hooked, represent 43% [33].

Intrinsic factors are the various processes that exist inside the rotator cuff itself. The most common of them is the degenerative-microtrauma model, which indicates that age-related tendon deterioration exacerbated by continuing microtrauma is the root cause of partial tendon tears that eventually transform into massive rotator cuff tears. After tearing, the deep fibers generally retract because they remain under stress even when the arm is relaxed. This results in greater stress on the remaining fibers, raising the risk of additional rupture. When a rotator cuff tendon is deteriorating, oxidative stress induces tenocyte death, which further deteriorates the tendon, and inflammatory mediators affect the local environment as a consequence of repeated microtrauma [33].

4.1.1 Physical therapy management

Below is a proposed five-phase rehabilitation protocol for patients undergoing rotator cuff repair, which is customized based on the size of the tear and the condition of the tendon tissue, which is consistent with recent studies and guidelines from the American Academy of Orthopedic Surgeons (AAOS) and the American Society of Shoulder and Elbow Therapists (ASSET) (**Figure 5**; **Table 2**) [35, 37].

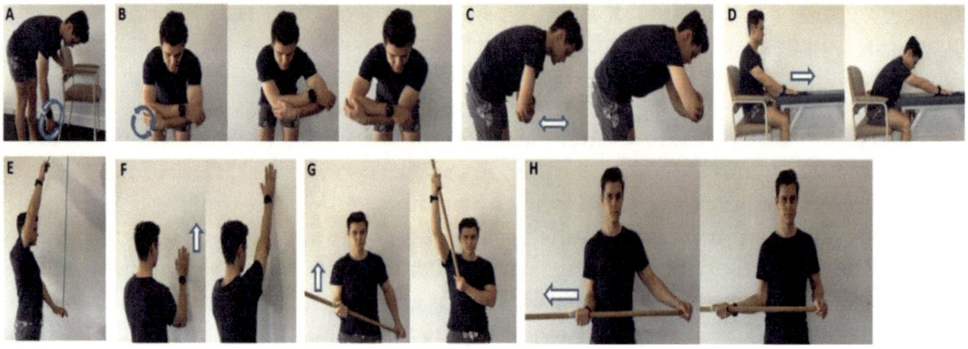

Figure 5.
Exercises for rotator cuff tears [34].

Phase 1	Complete immobilization (weeks 0–2). Active movement of the wrist and distal hand is permitted
Phase 2	Continued immobilization (weeks 2–6). The patient begins a protected PROM in the plane of the scapula. With the arm at the side, the elbow's active AROM is permitted. Under supervised physical therapy, it is possible to transition from PROM to an AAROM in weeks four through six. The following requirements must be met in order to proceed to the next stage—forward flexion or more than 120°, external rotation of more than 30°, and without pain PROM.
Phase 3	Weeks 6–12—Able to move from AAROM to AROM with a supraspinatus electromyographic activity rating of fewer than 15%. Complete and painless PROM and AROM with no compensation, no shoulder shrugging and painless isometric exercises are necessities for progression.
Phase 4	Weeks 12–20 endurance as well as strength with a supraspinatus electromyographic rating of 30–49%.
Phase 5	Weeks 20–26 strengthening of supraspinatus with electromyographic levels of activity above fifty percent [36].

Table 2.
Five-phase rehabilitation protocol for rotator cuff injury [35].

4.1.2 Pain management

The use of acetaminophen and NSAIDs is recommended for short-term pain relief in patients with rotator cuff injury. Any patient with severe pain or a contraindication to the above medication may be recommended short-term use of opioids for pain relief by a clinician. Corticosteroid injections, platelet-rich plasma injections (PRP), and hyaluronic injections for the reduction of pain and disability can be recommended by a clinician but not as a first-line measure [38].

4.2 Shoulder impingement syndrome

4.2.1 Physical therapy management

Impingement syndrome is a particular pathologic disease wherein the tendon of the supraspinatus experiences irritation due to friction against the anterior third part of the acromion's under surface [39].

Shoulder impingement syndrome can be classified based on the underlying etiology of the impingement (primary or secondary impingement) or the location of the impingement (internal or external). The soft tissue inside the subacromial space can either physically or mechanically intrude, causing external or subacromial impingement. On the contrary, internal impingement takes place when the rotator cuff's tendons infiltrate between the glenoid rim and humeral head. Most frequently, internal impingement is connected to the supraspinatus as well as the infraspinatus tendons.

Special tests are used to diagnose shoulder impingement syndrome. When used in combination, the Jobe test, Neer sign, the Hawkins test, and a painful arc of motion can define the picture of shoulder impingement syndrome, even though each test has limited sensitivity and specificity on its own (**Figures 6** and 7) [42].

With the goal of developing an organized conservative treatment plan, given below is a program that integrates manual therapy, stretching, strengthening, and education from multiple research studies [43–50].

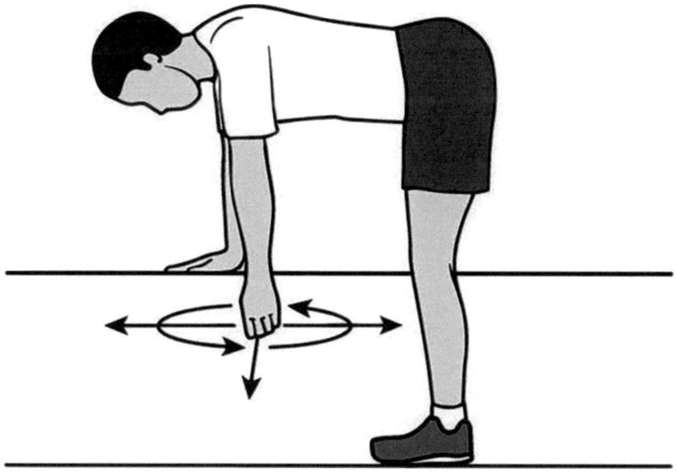

Figure 6.
Pendulum exercise [40].

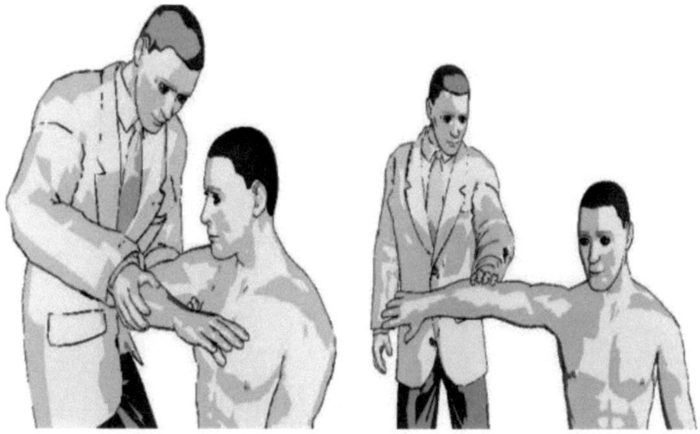

Figure 7.
Hawkins Kennedy and Jobe's test [41].

4.2.1.1 Acute phase, phase 1 (0–2 weeks)

Objectives: Improve scapular knowledge, restore pain-free range of motion, and minimize pain and inflammation.

1. Stretching:

- Stretching the pectoralis minor (corner stretch)—Place the forearms on either side of you while you stand in a doorway. Gently tilt forward, maintain the stretch for 30 seconds, repeat five times.

- Stretching the posterior shoulders (cross-body adduction)—Pull the afflicted arm over the chest five times, maintaining it for 30 seconds.

2. Painless ROM and Codman's pendulum exercises:

- Make little clockwise and anticlockwise circles while bending forward and allowing your arm to hang. Two sets of 10 repetitions, 2 times a day.

- Towel/cane-assisted range of motion—For passive flexion as well as external rotation, utilize a cane to internally rotate the arm behind the back, utilize a towel.

3. The modalities:

- Heat/ice packs (depending on inflammation)—15 minutes after exercising.

- If recommended, ultrasound or iontophoresis for pain reduction and improvement of ROM (**Figures 8** and **9**).

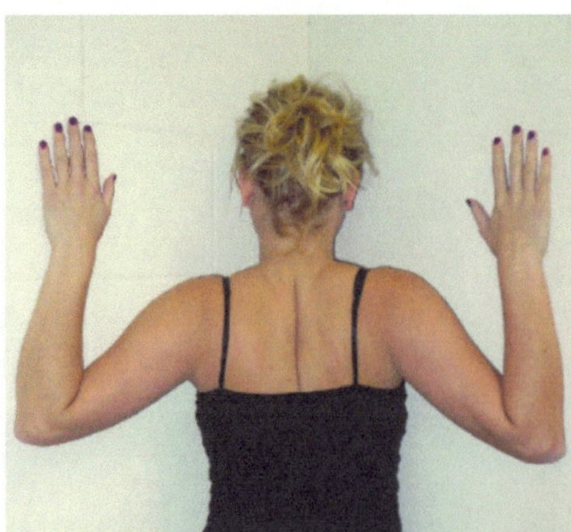

Figure 8.
Corner stretch [51].

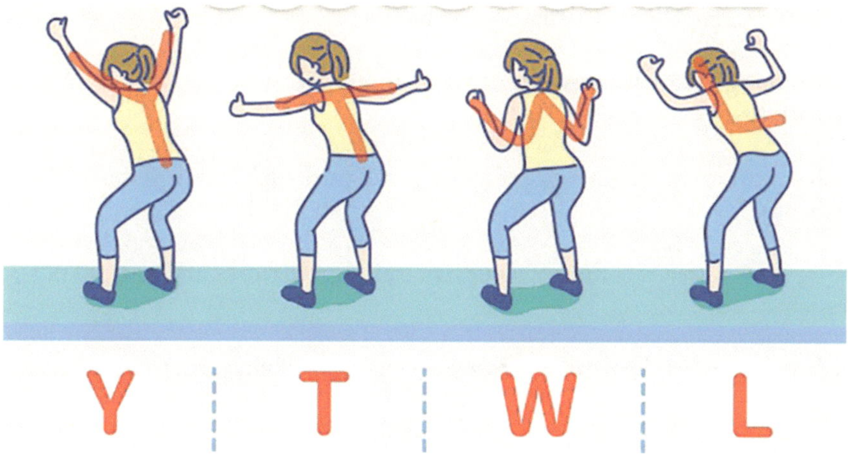

Figure 9.
YTWL exercises [52].

4.2.1.2 Intermediate phase, phase 2 (2 to 6 weeks)

Objectives: Enhance neuromuscular control as well as strengthen muscles of the rotator cuff and the muscles that stabilize the scapula.

1. Strength training (high repetitions, small resistance)

- Isometric rotator cuff exercise: push against a wall both when the shoulder is in internal rotation and external rotation, hold this for 5 seconds, and repeat 10 times.

- Stabilization of the scapula: scapular protraction (Supine): use a light weight when pushing arms upward.

- Scaption as well as rows: perform three sets with elastic bands of 10 repetitions.

2. Manual therapy

- Joint mobilization using the Maitland technique for inferior/anterior glides.

- Supraspinatus deep tissue massage for soft tissue release.

3. Adjusting posture

- During relaxation of the upper trapezius, mirrored feedback is provided to prevent the shrugging of shoulders.

- Foam rollers used during stretching for thoracic extension.

4.2.1.3 Advanced phase, phase 3 (6+ weeks)

Objectives: restarting activity, functional strength, as well as endurance.

1. Dynamic strengthening using elastic bands

- Maintaining external rotation at 0° and abduction at 90° perform 3 sets of 12 repetitions.
- Push-up progress: begin by performing wall push-ups, then advance to knee push-ups.

2. Using PNF patterns for proprioceptive training: rotator cuff hold-relax approaches.

- Assistive-resisted dynamic holds are an example of rhythmic stabilization.

3. Pectoral muscle/posterior shoulder routine stretching as a component of the home exercise.

- Body weight exercises and use of band for strengthening three times a week (**Figure 10**) [43–50].

4.2.2 Pain management

Tendinopathies have traditionally been managed by steroid injections. They could still, however, worsen the damaged tendon's potential to heal and promote tendon atrophy. Furthermore, research has indicated that steroid injections alone are not very effective. Growth hormones, along with other cytokines present in platelet-rich plasma (PRP), an enhanced platelet blood plasma, help to reinforce the body's healing response. Regardless of the fact that PRP injections are often used to treat tendon disorders, Foster et al.'s systematic review of the literature discovered that there is a lack of many controlled clinical studies that have effectively determined both the safety and efficacy of treatments. They reached a

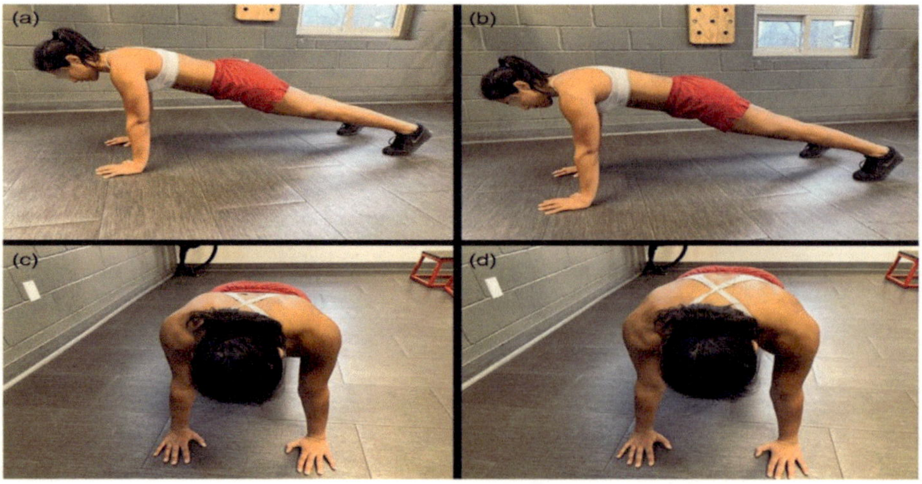

Figure 10.
Push Up [53].

verdict that PRP is a promising but untested alternative therapy for tendon as well as muscle injuries [38, 54].

4.3 Rotator cuff tendinopathy

A degenerative condition referred to as rotator cuff tendinopathy impacts the tendons attached to the rotator cuff muscles. It is often brought on by aging, repetitive overhead motions, or abnormalities in anatomical structure, such as a hooked acromion. Tendon integrity becomes compromised by this tendinopathy, leaving them susceptible to partial or full-thickness tears. As these tears get worse, they can affect the shoulder's biomechanics, leading the humeral head to shift superiorly and the subacromial space to narrow down. Subacromial impingement is a consequence of the aforementioned space restriction, which compresses the tendons as well as the bursa when the arm is elevated. Impingement causes the tendon injury to worsen, which reinforces the cycle of dysfunction and pain. If not treated, this progression from tendinopathy to tear and further impingement can significantly affect shoulder functioning [55].

Acromiohumeral distance, along with subacromial space, can be assessed with diagnostic ultrasound, which is a viable and efficient technique. Rehabilitation might be able to rectify the subacromial space reduction that develops after arm elevation in approximately 45% of patients with RC tendinopathy. Research on the impacts of RC muscle fatigue suggests that people with RC tendinopathy take a while to return to normal condition and that the subacromial space shrinks following fatigue. Furthermore, electromyography studies among individuals with RC tendinopathy demonstrated a delay in activation of the muscles controlling scapular movement and posture, as well as diminished RC muscle activation [56].

4.3.1 Physical therapy management

Exercise therapy is the first step in treatment. Strongest evidence is present for eccentric strengthening:

- Slow lowering phase of external rotation using Theraband or cable.
- Eccentric external rotation while side-lying (for 3–4 seconds, lowering the arm from 90° abduction).
- Performed five times a week, 3 sets of 15 repetitions.

(For acute pain) isometrics:

- Submaximal external rotation or internal rotation holds at 0° of abduction five times for 45 sec.

Additional interventions

- Manual therapy: Grade III–IV posterior capsule mobilizations to alleviate stiffness.

- Soft tissue release for the infraspinatus or teres minor muscle.
- To manage dyskinesia, prone Y/T/W exercises and rows are performed to help stabilize the scapula [57, 58].

The treatment for rotator cuff tendinopathy resembles early-stage treatment for impingement syndrome as seen in the treatment of impingement above (**Figure 11**).

4.4 Adhesive capsulitis

A common but not very well understood disorder, which leads to shoulder pain and limitation in range of motion, is adhesive capsulitis. It may manifest either by itself or in combination with diabetes mellitus or other shoulder disorders (e.g., bursitis or rotator cuff tendinopathy). A painful stage, a freezing stage, and a thawing or healing stage are the three consecutive stages of adhesive capsulitis. However, this classification has not been backed by any research, and its clinical relevance is dubious. Every phase of adhesive capsulitis, which typically fails to progress in a progressive manner, may lead to pain and a limited range of motion. Up to 10% of patients never restore their full range of motion, and pain and diminished range of motion may persist for as long as 2 years [59].

Adhesive capsulitis should be considered if there is a reduction of mobility with forward flexion, abduction, along with external and internal rotations. To accurately assess deficiencies, it is crucial to compare these movements on the afflicted and unaffected sides. To guarantee a precise assessment of movement, the patient must initially be requested to actively test their range of motion. If a loss of motion becomes apparent, the doctor may passively assist with scapular stability. The Apley scratch test, which is typically described in terms of the most significant vertebral level achieved, is the most commonly employed technique for determining internal

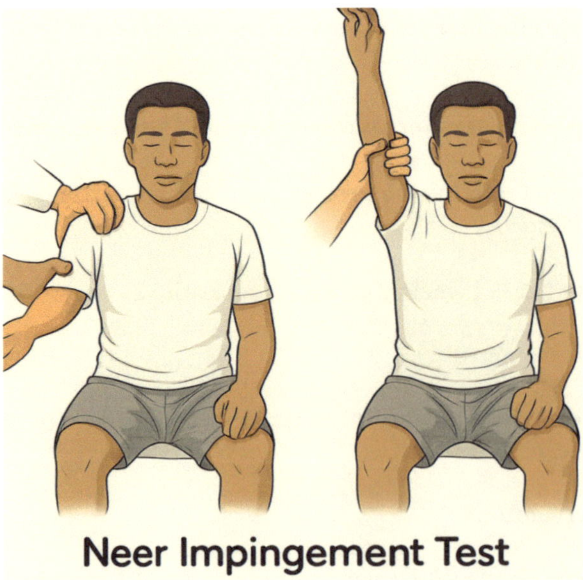

Figure 11.
Neer test (AI generated).

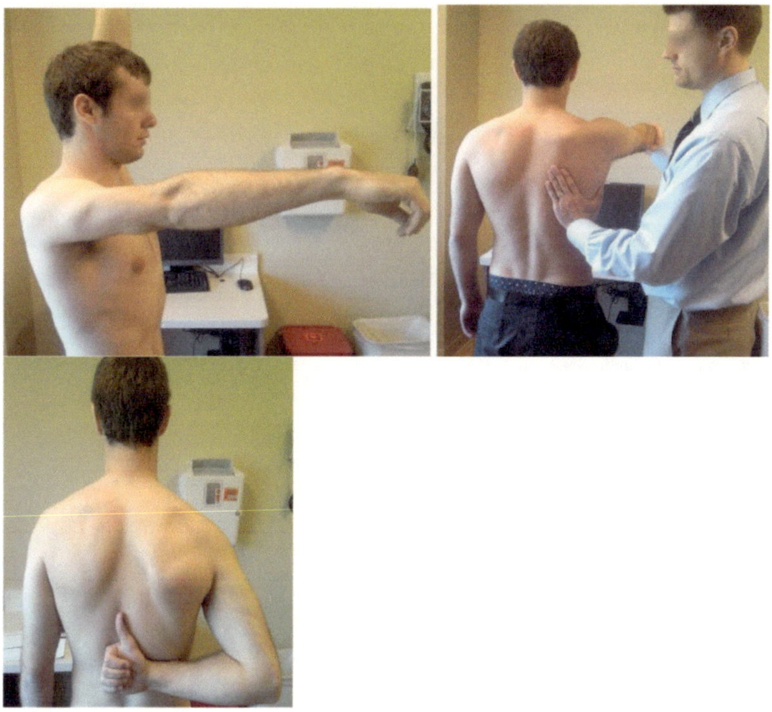

Figure 12.
Tests for adhesive capsulitis [60].

rotation. Any plane with a full range of motion points to a different diagnosis (**Figure 12**) [60].

4.4.1 Physical therapy management

4.4.1.1 Manual therapy

- Joint mobilizations (Maitland, Kaltenborn): Early-stage Grade I–II oscillations (pain management).

- Inferior/posterior glides, called Grade III–IV mobilizations, are used to increase capsular elasticity.

- When coupled with exercise, High-Grade Mobilizations (HGM) substantially improve a range of motion (Jain et al.).

- Soft tissue mobilization: Reducing stiffness in the pectoral as well as scapulothoracic regions (**Table 3**; **Figure 13**).

4.4.1.2 Pain management

- Cryotherapy and heat: For pain relief, apply heat before therapy and ice following therapy.

Phase 1 (Acute/painful stage)	• Gravity-assisted range of motion exercises using a pendulum (Codman's).
	• Using a pulley for flexion/abduction, or a therapist assisting in passive stretching.
Phase 2 (Stiffness dominates in this stage)	• AAROM (wall crawls, wand exercises)
	• Crossbody and sleeper stretches, which are capsular stretches
Phase 3	• Internal and external rotation using a Theraband for rotator cuff strengthening in the third phase, which is the recovery stage.
	• Prone Y/T/W exercises and rows for scapular stabilization.

Table 3.
Exercise therapy protocol for adhesive capsulitis [61].

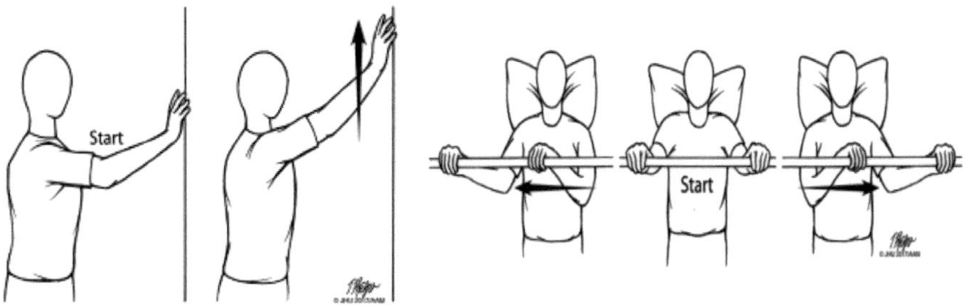

Figure 13.
Exercises for adhesive capsulitis [62].

- TENS and ultrasound have little evidence, but they may assist with the pain management.
- NSAIDs: Used for pain management.

4.4.1.3 Additional therapies

- Corticosteroids in the form of injections: Brief pain reduction (PT should begin in 2 to 4 weeks).
- When combined with PT, hydrodilatation (capsular distension) boosts results [63].

4.5 Shoulder instability

Excess translation by the humeral head inside the glenoid fossa causes shoulder instability, which may culminate in discomfort, subluxation, as well as dislocation. Traumatic damage (such as falling on an outstretched arm can cause anterior dislocation) or repetitive microtrauma (frequent in athletes with overhead activities) is the principal mechanism. Bankart lesions (labrum detachment) and capsular laxity are typical examples of structural damage, whereas neuromuscular dysfunctions can result in functional instability (rotator cuff weakness, scapular dyskinesia). Because of inadequate dynamic stabilizers (muscle coordination) and static stabilizers (ligaments/

labrum), persistent instability is common, particularly in young individuals. The MRI/ arthroscopy and the apprehension test assist in diagnosis affirmation [64].

4.5.1 Physical therapy management

4.5.1.1 Acute phase, stage 1 (0: 4 weeks)

Objectives: Preserve healing tissues and decrease pain, along with inflammation.
Interventions:

- Relative rest (avoid exacerbating positions, sling for ease).
- Isometrics (submaximal contractions of the scapula as well as the rotator cuff).
- Pendulum exercises (gravity-assisted range of motion).
- Pain relief methods include TENS and cryotherapy.

4.5.1.2 Intermediary period, stage 2 (4–12 Weeks)

- Objectives: restore neuromuscular control as well as dynamic stability.
- Interventions include progressive strengthening of rotator cuff external and internal rotators, as well as scapular stabilizers.
- Variations of plank and wall push-ups, which are closed-chain exercises.

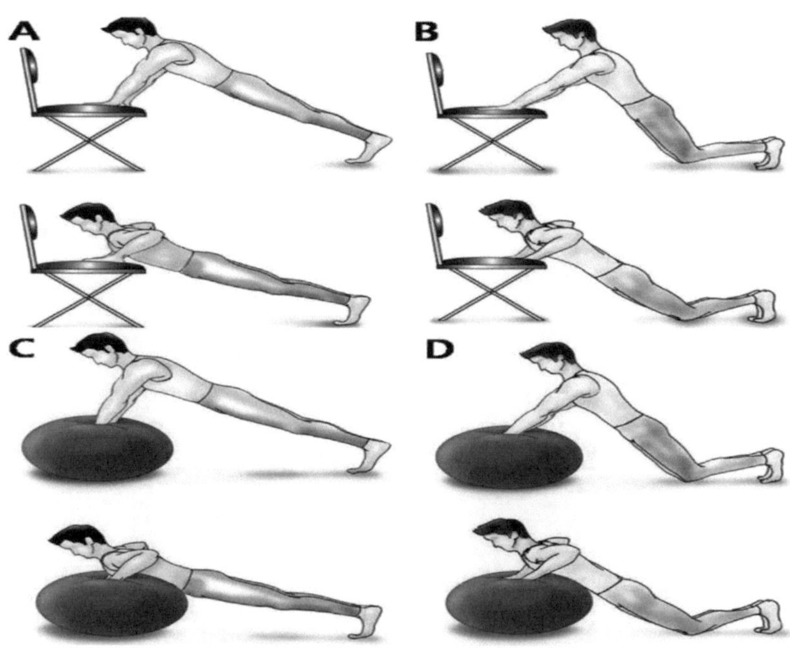

Figure 14.
Push Up progression [65].

- Exercises to improve proprioception (unstable surface training, PNF patterns).

4.5.1.3 Advanced, stage 3 (12+ Weeks)

- Rehab customized for a sport or activity and recurrence avoidance are the goals.
- Plyometric exercises (resisted rotations, ball throws).
- Overhead stabilization using kettlebell carries.
- Drills customized for a particular sport (gradual return to contact or throw) (**Figure 14**) [66].

4.6 Labral tears

Shoulder pain and instability are frequently brought on by glenoid labrum tears, which were formerly classified into anterior (Bankart), posterior (Reverse bankart), as well as superior labral tears (SLAP). A history obtained as part of the diagnostic process for labral tears pays special attention to clicking, shoulder instability, as well as pain during overhead activities. Apprehension, load and shift, inferior sulcus sign, and relocation, along with crank tests, were each component of the physical examination. MRI and shoulder arthroscopy can be used; however, physical examination is a more accurate predictor of glenoid labral tears than MRI [67, 68].

4.6.1 Physical therapy management

4.6.1.1 Non-operational management

- Top prospects: Partial tear, particularly type I or II SLAP.
- Athletes who do not perform overhead activities.
- Lack of mechanical signs, such as locking (**Figures 15** and **16**)

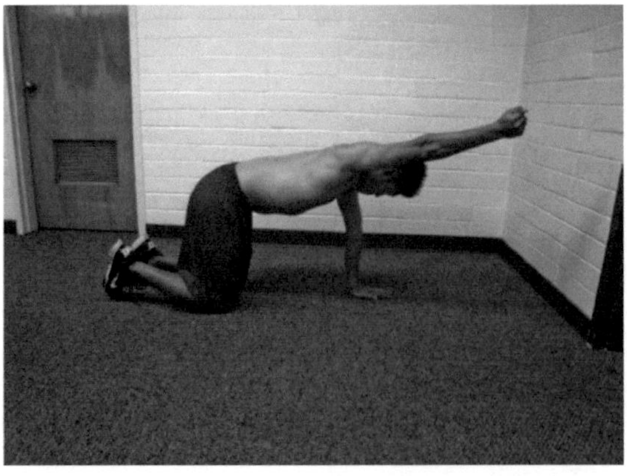

Figure 15.
Quadruped drills [69].

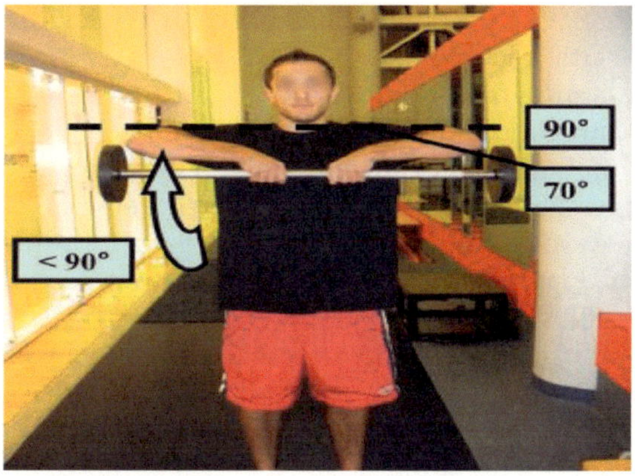

Figure 16.
Upright row [70].

Phase 1 (Weeks 1–6)	• Use ice as well as modify activity to decrease inflammation
	• Scapular stabilization through quadruped drills and rows.
	• Isometric activation of the rotator cuff
Phase 2 (Weeks 6–12)	• Eccentric strengthening of external and internal rotators at 45° abduction.
	• Progressively increase ROM while avoiding the 90/90 external/internal rotation position

Table 4.
Physical therapy protocol for labral tears [71].

The physical therapy protocol (**Table 4**):

Indications for surgery:

- Overhead athletes with type II–IV SLAP tears.
- Bankart lesions with recurring instability.
- PT failure: no improvement even after 3–6 months.

Rehabilitation following surgery

- Bankart lesion repair: 4 weeks of immobilization preceding gradual range of motion, external rotation will be restricted for up to the 6th week.
- SLAP lesion repair: 8 to 12 weeks of no active bicep loading.
- Overhead movements are delayed for up to 12 weeks.

5. Conclusion

The shoulder joint is especially prone to damage and dysfunction because of its extensive range of motion and intricate anatomical structure. The anatomy and biomechanics of the shoulder complex have been thoroughly covered in this chapter, with special attention paid to the delicate balance between stability and mobility that is preserved by both static and dynamic structures.

We discussed the clinical manifestations, diagnostic methods, and underlying pathophysiology of common shoulder diseases, including tendinopathy, adhesive capsulitis, shoulder impingement syndrome, rotator cuff tears, and various types of instability. In-depth evaluation techniques were also covered in order to help physicians correctly diagnose and distinguish between shoulder disorders.

An evidence-based approach to rehabilitation, with well-defined procedures catered to particular illnesses and stages of recovery, was at the heart of this chapter. In order to restore function, lessen pain, and stop recurrence, these included manual therapy, therapeutic exercises, neuromuscular re-education, and pain management techniques.

This chapter is a useful tool for physicians, physical therapists, and students working on shoulder diseases since it combines in-depth anatomical information with the clinical best practices. Optimizing patient outcomes and fostering functional rehabilitation need a deep comprehension and implementation of these concepts.

Acknowledgements

We would like to express our sincere gratitude to the Department of Rehabilitation Sciences at The University of Faisalabad for providing academic support and resources essential for the development of this chapter. Special thanks to our mentors and colleagues whose guidance and critical insights enriched the quality and depth of this work. Finally, we thank IntechOpen for the opportunity to contribute to this scholarly publication and for fostering a platform that promotes the dissemination of evidence-based knowledge to the global scientific and medical community. The author acknowledges the use of ChatGPT for language polishing of the manuscript as well as the preparation of **Figure 11**.

Conflict of interest

No conflict of interest.

Notes/thanks/other declarations

We want to express our gratitude to the physiotherapy community and all other professionals who work tirelessly to improve patient care by using evidence-based practice and clinical research. The ongoing quest for perfection in musculoskeletal rehabilitation and practical clinical issues served as inspiration for the creation of this chapter. This chapter's exercises, protocols, and interventions are based on current research as well as clinical experience. Practitioners are encouraged to modify the material, nevertheless, in light of changing research, clinical judgment, and the needs of specific patients.

Nomenclature

GH Joint (glenohumeral joint)	a ball-and-socket synovial joint between the head of the humerus and the glenoid cavity of the scapula.

SC Joint (sternoclavicular joint)	a saddle-type joint between the sternum and clavicle.
AC Joint (acromioclavicular joint)	a plane joint between the acromion of the scapula and the clavicle.
SLAP lesion	superior labral anterior to posterior tear in the glenoid labrum.
Bankart lesion	a tear of the labrum due to anterior shoulder dislocation.
SITS muscles	supraspinatus, infraspinatus, teres minor, subscapularis—components of the rotator cuff.
PROM	passive range of motion—movement performed by the therapist without patient effort.
AROM	active range of motion—patient moves joint without assistance.
AAROM	active-assisted range of motion—movement assisted by therapist or equipment.
ROM	range of motion—the extent of movement of a joint.
PRP	platelet-rich plasma—blood plasma enriched with platelets, used in regenerative therapy.
NSAIDs	non-steroidal anti-inflammatory drugs—medications used to reduce inflammation and pain.

A. Special tests for shoulder evaluation

See **Table A1.**

Test	Purpose	Associated condition
Neer test	Impingement	Shoulder impingement syndrome
Hawkins-Kennedy test	Impingement	Subacromial impingement
Jobe's test	Supraspinatus integrity	Rotator cuff tear
Speed's test	Biceps tendon pathology	Bicipital tendinitis
Apprehension test	Instability	Anterior shoulder instability
Sulcus sign	Inferior laxity	Shoulder subluxation
Crank test	Labral tear detection	SLAP lesion, Bankart lesion
Apley scratch test	ROM assessment	Adhesive capsulitis

Table A1.

B. Rehabilitation protocol overview

See **Table A2.**

Phase	Goal	Key interventions
Phase 1	Immobilization and pain control	Passive ROM, pendulum exercises, cryotherapy
Phase 2	Protected mobilization	PROM → AAROM, scapular control, isometrics
Phase 3	Strengthening	AROM, rotator cuff strengthening, posture correction
Phase 4	Advanced strength and endurance	Resistance bands, proprioceptive training
Phase 5	Return to function	Plyometric drills, sport-specific training

Table A2.

Author details

Adeera Azam[1*], Ishal Ayub[1], Lyba Musaddiq[2], Esha Dilawar[1] and Muhammad Suleman Tahir[3]

1 The University of Faisalabad, Pakistan

2 Faisalabad Institute of Management and Sciences, Faisalabad, Pakistan

3 Anam Rehab and the Physio Lab, Pakistan

*Address all correspondence to: adeeraazam.dpt@tuf.edu.pk

References

[1] Kadi R, Milants A, Shahabpour M. Shoulder anatomy and normal variants. Journal of the Belgian Society of Radiology. 2017;**101**(Suppl 2):3

[2] Flores DV, Goes PK, Gómez CM, Umpire DF, Pathria MN. Imaging of the acromioclavicular joint: Anatomy, function, pathologic features, and treatment. Radiographics. 2020;**40**(5):1355-1382

[3] Bigliani LU, Kelkar R, Flatow EL, Pollock RG, Mow VC. Glenohumeral stability: Biomechanical properties of passive and active stabilizers. Clinical Orthopaedics and Related Research (1976-2007). 1996;**330**:13-30

[4] Verma N. Shoulder Anatomy | Shoulder Injuries | Chicago Westchester Oakbrook Hinsdale IL [Internet]. Chicago: Midwest Orthopaedics at Rush

[5] Chang L-R, Anand P, Varacallo MA. Anatomy, Shoulder and Upper Limb, Glenohumeral Joint. Treasure Island (FL): StatPearls Publishing; 2023

[6] Clavert P. Glenoid labrum pathology. Orthopaedics & Traumatology: Surgery & Research. 2015;**101**(1):S19-S24

[7] Chen J, Phadnis J. Glenohumeral capsule and ligaments. Normal and Pathological Anatomy of the Shoulder. 2015;**1**:93-99

[8] Bosson A, Ward K, Horsley I. The shoulder region: Anatomy, assessment and injuries. In: Routledge Handbook of Sports Therapy, Injury Assessment and Rehabilitation. London, New York: Routledge; 2015. pp. 366-441

[9] Cuéllar R, Ruiz-Ibán MA, Cuéllar A. Anatomy and biomechanics of the unstable shoulder. The Open Orthopaedics Journal. 2017;**11**:919

[10] Seth A, Matias R, Veloso AP, Delp SL. A biomechanical model of the scapulothoracic joint to accurately capture scapular kinematics during shoulder movements. PLoS One. 2016;**11**(1):e0141028

[11] Kock A. Shoulder Anatomy. Bursae and Muscles. Vector Illustration [Internet]. Adobe Stock

[12] Yang S, Kim TU, Kim DH, Chang MC. Understanding the physical examination of the shoulder: A narrative review. Annals of Palliative Medicine. 2021;**10**(2):2293303-2292303

[13] Itoi E, Hsu H-C, An K-N. Biomechanical investigation of the glenohumeral joint. Journal of Shoulder and Elbow Surgery. 1996;**5**(5):407-424

[14] Allen H, Chan BY, Davis KW, Blankenbaker DG. Overuse injuries of the shoulder. Radiologic Clinics. 2019;**57**(5):897-909

[15] Horowitz EH, Aibinder WR. Shoulder impingement syndrome. Physical Medicine and Rehabilitation Clinics. 2023;**34**(2):311-334

[16] Garving C, Jakob S, Bauer I, Nadjar R, Brunner UH. Impingement syndrome of the shoulder. Deutsches Ärzteblatt International. 2017;**114**(45):765

[17] Fell I, Tashjian RZ, Schroeder NS. Shoulder injuries. In: Orthopaedic Rotations Survival Guide. Philadelphia (PA): Wolters Kluwer; 2023

[18] Warth RJ, Millett PJ. Physical Examination of the Shoulder. Cham, Switzerland: Springer; 2015

[19] Finucane L, Mercer C, Hepburn A, Rajasekaran R, Cosker T. Red flags, inflammatory conditions and sinister shoulder pathology. In: The Shoulder: Theory and Practice. 1st ed. London: Handspring Publishing; 2022. pp. 99-111

[20] Bradford J. Subacromial Impingement Syndrome: Biomechanics, Pathology, Diagnosis, and Treatment. Chapel Hill, NC, USA: UNC; 2018

[21] Dougherty J, Walmsley S, Osmotherly PG. Passive range of movement of the shoulder: A standardized method for measurement and assessment of intrarater reliability. Journal of Manipulative and Physiological Therapeutics. 2015;**38**(3):218-224

[22] Pandey R, Raval P, Manibanakar N, Nanjayan S, McDonald C, Singh H. Proximal humerus fractures: A review of current practice. Journal of Clinical Orthopaedics and Trauma. 2023;**43**:102233

[23] Physiotutors. Speed's Test Illustration [Internet]

[24] Iyer KM. Clinical examination of the shoulder (basic and surface anatomy) with special tests. In: Orthopedics of the Upper and Lower Limb. Springer; 2020

[25] Fieseler G, Schwesig R, Sendler J, Cornelius J, Schulze S, Lehmann W, et al. IRO/shift test is comparable to the Jobe test for detection of supraspinatus lesions. Journal of Personalized Medicine. 2022;**12**(9):1422

[26] Verweij LP, Baden DN, van der Zande JM, van den Bekerom MP. Assessment and management of shoulder dislocation. BMJ. 2020;**371**:m4485

[27] Lizzio VA, Meta F, Fidai M, Makhni EC. Clinical evaluation and physical exam findings in patients with anterior shoulder instability. Current Reviews in Musculoskeletal Medicine. 2017;**10**:434-441

[28] Burton RJ, Barnard AR, Copas D, Talbot C. Neurovascular injury in shoulder girdle trauma. Orthopaedics and Traumatology. 2023;**37**(5):276-284

[29] De Filippo M, Schirò S, Sarohia D, Barile A, Saba L, Cella S, et al. Imaging of shoulder instability. Skeletal Radiology. 2020;**49**:1505-1523

[30] Sebelego I-K. Radiographers' utilisation of Radiographic Critique of Routine Shoulder Projections. Bloemfontein: Central University of Technology, Free State; 2016

[31] Feuerriegel GC, Weiss K, Van AT, Leonhardt Y, Neumann J, Gassert FT, et al. Deep-learning-based image quality enhancement of CT-like MR imaging in patients with suspected traumatic shoulder injury. European Journal of Radiology. 2024;**170**:111246

[32] Craig R, Holt T, Rees JL. Acute rotator cuff tears. BMJ. 2017;**359**:j5366

[33] Yadav H, Nho S, Romeo A, MacGillivray JD. Rotator cuff tears: Pathology and repair. Knee Surgery, Sports Traumatology, Arthroscopy. 2009;**17**:409-421

[34] Edwards PK, Kwong PWH, Ackland T, Wang A, Donnelly CJ, Ebert JR. Electromyographic evaluation of early-stage shoulder rehabilitation exercises following rotator cuff repair. International Journal of Sports Physical Therapy. 2021;**16**(6):1459-1469

[35] Longo UG, Risi Ambrogioni L, Berton A, Candela V, Migliorini F, Carnevale A, et al. Conservative versus accelerated rehabilitation after rotator

cuff repair: A systematic review and meta-analysis. BMC Musculoskeletal Disorders. 2021;**22**:1-22

[36] Sciarretta FV, Moya D, List K. Current trends in rehabilitation of rotator cuff injuries. Sicot Journal. 2023;**9**:14

[37] Mazuquin B, Moffatt M, Gill P, Selfe J, Rees J, Drew S, et al. Effectiveness of early versus delayed rehabilitation following rotator cuff repair: Systematic review and meta-analyses. PLoS One. 2021;**16**(5):e0252137

[38] Desmeules F, Roy J-S, Lafrance S, Charron M, Dubé M-O, Dupuis F, et al. Rotator cuff tendinopathy diagnosis, non-surgical medical care and rehabilitation: A clinical practice guideline. Journal of Orthopaedic & Sports Physical Therapy. 2025;**55**(3):1-94

[39] Morrison DS, Greenbaum BS, Einhorn A. Shoulder impingement. Orthopedic Clinics of North America. 2000;**31**(2):285-293

[40] Mobile Physiotherapy Clinic. Deltoid Muscle Exercise [Internet]

[41] Tennent TD, Beach WR, Meyers JF. A review of the special tests associated with shoulder examination: Part I: The rotator cuff tests. The American Journal of Sports Medicine. 2003;**31**(1):154-160

[42] Cools AM, Cambier D, Witvrouw EE. Screening the athlete's shoulder for impingement symptoms: A clinical reasoning algorithm for early detection of shoulder pathology. British Journal of Sports Medicine. 2008;**42**(8):628-635

[43] Yemul SR. Comparison of supervised exercise with and without manual physical therapy for patients with shoulder impingement syndrome. International Journal of Current Research and Review. 2013;**5**(5):144

[44] Brox JI, Gjengedal E, Uppheim G, Bøhmer AS, Brevik JI, Ljunggren AE, et al. Arthroscopic surgery versus supervised exercises in patients with rotator cuff disease (stage II impingement syndrome): A prospective, randomized, controlled study in 125 patients with a 212-year follow-up. Journal of Shoulder and Elbow Surgery. 1999;**8**(2):102-111

[45] Conroy DE, Hayes KW. The effect of joint mobilization as a component of comprehensive treatment for primary shoulder impingement syndrome. Journal of Orthopaedic & Sports Physical Therapy. 1998;**28**(1):3-14

[46] Haahr JP, Østergaard S, Dalsgaard J, Norup K, Frost P, Lausen S, et al. Exercises versus arthroscopic decompression in patients with subacromial impingement: A randomised, controlled study in 90 cases with a one year follow up. Annals of the Rheumatic Diseases. 2005;**64**(5):760-764

[47] Ludewig P, Borstad J. Effects of a home exercise programme on shoulder pain and functional status in construction workers. Occupational and Environmental Medicine. 2003;**60**(11):841-849

[48] Peters G, Kohn D. Medium-term clinical results after operative and non-operative treatment of subacromial impingement. Der Unfallchirurg. 1997;**100**:623-629

[49] Rahme H, Solem-Bertoft E, Westerberg C-E, Lundberg E, Sörensen S, Hilding S. The subacromial impingement syndrome. A study of results of treatment with special emphasis on predictive factors and pain-generating mechanisms. Scandinavian

Journal of Rehabilitation Medicine. 1998;**30**(4):253-262

[50] Senbursa G, Baltacı G, Atay A. Comparison of conservative treatment with and without manual physical therapy for patients with shoulder impingement syndrome: A prospective, randomized clinical trial. Knee Surgery, Sports Traumatology, Arthroscopy. 2007;**15**:915-921

[51] Durall C. Therapeutic exercise for athletes with nonspecific neck pain: A current concepts review. Sports Health. 2012;**4**:293-301

[52] Smith J, Lee R, Brown T. Scapular stabilization exercises: Y-T-W-L formation illustrations. Journal of Sports Medicine and Rehabilitation. 2023;**15**(2):123-126

[53] Kowalski KL, Connelly DM, Jakobi JM, Sadi J. Shoulder electromyography activity during push-up variations: A scoping review. Shoulder & Elbow. 2022;**14**(3):325-339

[54] Foster TE, Puskas BL, Mandelbaum BR, Gerhardt MB, Rodeo SA. Platelet-rich plasma: From basic science to clinical applications. The American Journal of Sports Medicine. 2009;**37**(11):2259-2272

[55] Factor D, Dale B. Current concepts of rotator cuff tendinopathy. International Journal of Sports Physical Therapy. 2014;**9**(2):274-288

[56] Lewis J, McCreesh K, Roy J-S, Ginn K. Rotator cuff tendinopathy: Navigating the diagnosis-management conundrum. Journal of Orthopaedic & Sports Physical Therapy. 2015;**45**(11):923-937

[57] Littlewood C, Ashton J, Chance-Larsen K, May S, Sturrock B. Exercise for rotator cuff tendinopathy: A systematic review. Physiotherapy. 2012;**98**(2):101-109

[58] Clinic MC. Y-W-T Exercises for Scapular Stabilisation. 2025. Available from: https://maristowchiropractic.com/uploads/exercises/ywt.pdf

[59] Hand G, Athanasou N, Matthews T, Carr A. The pathology of frozen shoulder. The Journal of Bone & Joint Surgery British Volume. 2007;**89**(7):928-932

[60] Ewald A. Adhesive capsulitis: A review. American Family Physician. 2011;**83**(4):417-422

[61] Miller MD, Wirth MA, Rockwood CA Jr. Thawing the frozen shoulder: The "patient" patient. Orthopedics. Oct 1996;**19**(10):915-920

[62] EG M, JL R, M B. Shoulder range of motion exercises2017 2025/05/17. Available from: https://cdn.ymaws.com/wichiro.org/resource/collection/53DBDFEA-02AA-4DFD-9698-6030F77041A2/Shoulder-rom_-_John_Hopkins_Series_incl._CANE_.pdf

[63] Jain TK, Sharma NK. The effectiveness of physiotherapeutic interventions in treatment of frozen shoulder/adhesive capsulitis: A systematic review. Journal of Back and Musculoskeletal Rehabilitation. 2014;**27**(3):247-273

[64] Farrar NG, Malal JJ, Fischer J, Waseem M. An overview of shoulder instability and its management. The Open Orthopaedics Journal. 2013;7:338-346

[65] Seo S-H, Jeon I-H, Cho Y-H, Lee H-G, Hwang Y-T, Jee HJ. Surface EMG during the push-up plus exercise on a stable support or Swiss ball: Scapular stabilizer muscle exercise.

Journal of Physical Therapy Science. 2013;**25**:833-837

[66] Jaggi A, Alexander S. Rehabilitation for shoulder instability - current approaches. The Open Orthopaedics Journal. 2017;**11**:957-971

[67] Alexeev M, Kercher JS, Levina Y, Duralde XA. Variability of glenoid labral tear patterns: A study of 280 sequential surgical cases. Journal of Shoulder and Elbow Surgery. 2021;**30**(12):2762-2766

[68] Liu SH, Henry MH, Nuccion S, Shapiro MS, Dorey F. Diagnosis of glenoid labral tears: A comparison between magnetic resonance imaging and clinical examinations. The American Journal of Sports Medicine. 1996;**24**(2):149-154

[69] Tsuruike M, Ellenbecker TS. Serratus anterior and lower trapezius muscle activities during multi-joint isotonic scapular exercises and isometric contractions. Journal of Athletic Training. 2015;**50**(2):199-210

[70] Schoenfeld B, Kolber M, Haimes J. The upright row: Implications for preventing subacromial impingement. Strength & Conditioning Journal. 2011;**33**:25-28

[71] Massachusetts General Brigham Sports Medicine. Rehabilitation Protocol for Superior Labrum Anterior and Posterior (SLAP) Repair [Internet]

Chapter 2

Perspective Chapter: Cervical Contribution in Shoulder Pain

Alberto Roldán-Ruiz and Gabriele Bertotti

Abstract

Shoulder pain is a prevalent musculoskeletal condition that might be influenced by the cervical spine, with this phenomenon being frequently overlooked in clinical assessments. This diagnosis could be named cervical contribution, and the intricate relationship between cervical pathologies and shoulder pain is underscored by various studies indicating that cervical structures may refer pain to the shoulder. This relationship highlights the importance of considering cervical contribution when diagnosing and treating shoulder pain, as traditional assessments may fail to account for these interdependencies. In clinical practice, the misdiagnosis of shoulder pain as purely shoulder-related, without considering cervical factors, can lead to ineffective treatment strategies and poor patient outcomes. Therefore, a comprehensive evaluation that includes cervical spine assessment is essential for accurate diagnosis and effective management of shoulder pain. This chapter aims to elucidate neurophysiological, biomechanical, and clinical reasoning supporting the cervical contribution to shoulder pain, advocating for a more integrative approach in clinical settings.

Keywords: shoulder pain, cervical contribution, cervical spine, diagnosis, physical therapy, clinical reasoning

1. Introduction

Shoulder pain diagnosis has historically followed a pathoanatomical perspective, distinguishing between intrinsic and extrinsic origins [1]. Although most shoulder discomfort might have an intrinsic origin (e.g., rotator cuff-related shoulder pain, acromioclavicular joint pain, biceps tendinopathy), the presence of referred pain from extrinsic structures may exist. Indeed, pain arising from the cervical and/or thoracic spine could also be considered an extrinsic entity. Besides this, referred pain could also constitute an indicator of more serious conditions [2].

Therefore, the presence of systemic symptoms such as fever, weight loss, and/or associated respiratory problems is a possible indicator of an extrinsic source of shoulder pain and, more specifically, of serious pathologies. For instance, pathological conditions such as myocardial ischemia, polymyalgia rheumatica, metastasis, apex lung cancer, pneumonia, or cervical nerve root compression could be the source of extrinsic shoulder pain [2, 3]. In this manner, the first step in managing a shoulder pain patient is ruling out serious pathology. This screening phase should not be regarded as trivial, and clinicians should take this into account.

1.1 Musculoskeletal shoulder pain

When having ruled out serious pathology and thus managing musculoskeletal shoulder pain, clinicians are still overusing unreliable orthopedic tests and imaging [4], when it might be the time to definitely abandon the pathoanatomic model in favor of the biopsychosocial model [5].

Therefore, musculoskeletal shoulder pain might involve nociceptive mechanism arising from peripheral structures (e.g., muscles, tendons, joints, ligaments, intervertebral discs), at least initially. Although this is a plausible explanation, it is not possible to confirm that the pain experienced by a person is caused by a particular structure, with a 100% probability.

In this context, it is known that pain is complex and multifactorial, so patients often describe musculoskeletal pain as diffuse, responding to on-and-off onset of pain and a more or less localized pain distribution, depending on the temporal stage. In these cases, peripheral and central sensitization mechanisms have been suggested that could play a significant role in its production and persistence [6]. In addition, this type of condition typically presents signs and symptoms in the deltoid area, arm, and scapular region. Common characteristics include stiffness and loss of mobility, often resulting in limitations in daily activities [7]. Additionally, pain usually changes with movement and/or rest and shoulder pain that symptomatically responds to postural changes or repeated movements may be considered mechanical in nature [8].

Nevertheless, in cases where central processing mechanisms are assessed and identified as predominant, the movement might not be as relevant as the patient's beliefs and attitudes regarding their pain. In musculoskeletal shoulder pain, similar to other conditions, these aspects can influence pain perpetuation and determine the ineffectiveness of certain treatments [9].

1.2 Shoulder pain subclassifications

Given the aforementioned, a paradigm shift in shoulder pain management, specifically in clinical reasoning and diagnosis, might be deemed necessary. As previously mentioned, due to the fact that pain experience is individual, multifactorial, and contextual [10, 11], the pathoanatomical model does not seem justified based on available scientific research [12, 13]. While diagnosis based on intrinsic and extrinsic aspects may help to understand the pathogenesis and etiology of shoulder pain by considering some biomechanical and neurophysiological interdependencies, it does not resolve all conditionings to achieve accurate diagnoses. Therefore, in order to overcome current difficulties with inter-examiner agreement in diagnosing shoulder pain, it may be necessary to rely on subclassifying patients with easily and validly reproducible common characteristics [14].

Throughout the years, various distinct subclassifications for shoulder pain have been suggested [15–18]. In 2005, Mitchell et al. suggested a clinical algorithm to classify shoulder pain, including diagnoses of referred pain from the cervical spine, shoulder instability, glenohumeral joint disorders, rotator cuff disorders, and acromioclavicular joint disease [3]. In 2014, another similar reasoning algorithm was proposed, including the same subgroups of cervical origin pain, instability, glenohumeral joint disorders, and rotator cuff tendinopathy [19]. Both classification systems identified rotator cuff pathology as the most diagnosed disorder. A similar approach has been reported lately, with the rotator cuff problems being the highest prevalent condition but closely followed by stiff shoulder problems and cervical contribution [20]. This agrees with other studies reporting that up to 85% of patients with shoulder pain showed rotator cuff tendinopathy [21]. Overall, it is possible that the high prevalence of findings related to rotator cuff pathology represents a key factor that has drawn the attention of both clinicians and researchers in a manner that other interconnections (e.g., cervical spine) have been overlooked.

When considering shoulder pain diagnosis and subclassification, the cervical contribution is a shoulder diagnosis that might encompass other terms that have been lately reported such as cervical origin or cervical derangement [22–27]. Furthermore, some authors argued that the cervical spine should be examined, and its involvement excluded, prior to any other specific shoulder diagnosis hypothesis [28–30].

2. Cervical contribution in shoulder pain

Although still limited, scientific literature regarding cervical contribution in shoulder pain is indeed experiencing a growing momentum, and it increasingly seems that this interregional influence may have a relevant role in shoulder pain management.

Considering the idea that the clinical decision-making process might be wrong if it fully relies on the anatomical region presenting symptoms [28, 30–32], it is worth noting that inadequate patient management may come from diagnosing a shoulder problem when in reality we do come across with a neck-related shoulder problem [25].

Building on this idea, some authors suggest that the cervical spine should be assessed first, and its involvement ruled out before establishing a specific shoulder diagnosis [28–30]. A recent Delphi study has attempted to establish a consensus on spine screening in patients with shoulder pain, incorporating strategies such as assessing changes in shoulder symptoms with neck movements or active cervical movements [33]. Even though new integrative approaches have been proposed [34], the most effective methods for screening the cervical spine in cases of shoulder pain have yet to be determined [35, 36].

In fact, since establishing a diagnosis based on the nociceptive source of symptoms currently seems not to be possible, this approach should be reserved for academic situations, while in clinical practice, principles of clinical reasoning based on symptomatic responses to mechanical stimuli during evaluation and treatment should be applied [8].

In this regard, it has been described that sustained or repeated cervical movements can modify shoulder pain, and if this is found as a significant finding during examination, cervical contribution can be considered a diagnostic hypothesis [8, 25].

In this manner, cervical contribution in shoulder pain should be comparable to what usually occurs in low back pain: to confirm sacroiliac involvement in low back pain, it is necessary to first rule out the lumbar origin so that sacroiliac tests can achieve high specificity. This has been studied in the presence of the centralization phenomenon, specific to discogenic pain [37]. In other words, if sacroiliac tests are performed in situations of discogenic referred pain, these tests might yield false positives, hence the need to first rule out discogenic pain to increase the diagnostic validity of sacroiliac tests is shown [37]. A similar scenario might occur in shoulder pain, as it has been described that shoulder-specific orthopedic tests may yield false-positive results in patients with shoulder pain when underlying spinal disorders remain undiagnosed [38]. Therefore, it might be necessary to first rule out cervical contribution when managing shoulder pain patients. And this is not only necessary in research for epidemiological studies but also to improve and guide interventions and prognosis within clinical practice scenario [8, 28, 30–32].

Regarding the cervical spine contribution in shoulder pain, there is no homogeneity in the used terms. About four observational studies found in the literature, two of them used the term 'cervical origin' [25, 26], one employed the term associated with The McKenzie system of Mechanical Diagnosis and Therapy (MDT), which is 'Spinal Derangement' or 'Cervical Spine Derangement' [24], and one used the 'Cervical Contribution' [34]. Similarly, other observational studies used terms like 'spinal contribution' to distal problems, referring to radiculopathy conditions associated with electromyographic changes [39] or radicular problems, for instance, radiculitis [40]. Regarding the actual diagnostic description in the first three mentioned studies, Karel et al. [26] did not define the criteria used to identify patients with shoulder problems originated from the cervical or thoracic region. Heidar Abady et al. and Rosedale et al. [24, 25] made a similar consideration, understanding a cervical diagnostic categorization as a positive symptom modification response exclusively associated with cervical spine treatment. Finally, Roldán-Ruiz et al. established that cervical contribution might be considered if a > 30% symptom modification occurred after neck approaches [34].

2.1 Spine and shoulder biomechanics

The biomechanical connection between the cervical spine and shoulder girdle suggests that dysfunction in cervical structures can lead to altered shoulder mechanics, thereby contributing to pain [41, 42]. In this context, the biomechanical relationship between the cervical spine and shoulder mobility remains largely unexplored. Only one study has investigated the mechanical response of the cervical spine during shoulder abduction, reporting that cervical vertebrae exhibited contralateral rotation up to 90° of shoulder abduction, with the greatest rotation occurring at the C6 vertebra (5.2°) [43].

Indeed, regarding shoulder and spine biomechanics, the thoracic spine has always been the region considered a key contributor to overhead movements [44], setting the cervical spine aside in this matter. Notably, individuals with subacromial impingement exhibit greater deficits in thoracic mobility within the sagittal and frontal planes compared to those without shoulder pathology [45, 46], with this being linked to increased thoracic kyphosis in individuals with this shoulder condition [47]. Similarly, patients with rotator cuff-related shoulder pain exhibit reduced thoracic spine flexion, extension, and rotational mobility compared to asymptomatic individuals [48].

2.2 Neck neuromuscular control and shoulder function

The relationship between upper limb movements and cervical neuromuscular control is justified by the feedforward systems, where muscular activity stabilizes the head and neck when upper limb movement is produced, and this process arises from the activity of deep neck flexors [49–51].

The interplay between neck function and shoulder pain is a complex, interconnected relationship where changes in one component may influence the others.

Observational studies have highlighted this association, such as research on elite handball players, which found a significant correlation ($r = -0.70$, $p = 0.02$) between cervical motor control dysfunction—identified through the craniocervical flexion test—and shoulder pain [52].

Additionally, improvements in neck pain have been observed following interventions focused on scapular positioning, emphasizing the role of axioscapular muscles in cervical function [53]. Moreover, studies indicate that repeated sagittal plane cervical movements can enhance cervical muscle function, as assessed by the craniocervical flexion test, suggesting a link between cervical joint integrity and muscle performance [54].

Given these findings, it is plausible that cervical neuromuscular control influences upper limb movement. A potential explanation for this is that deficits in deep cervical flexor muscles may contribute to suboptimal baseline conditions for upper limb mobility, leading to non-optimal movement patterns. This supports the possibility of a bidirectional interaction between cervical and shoulder function concerning neuromuscular control. However, while these associations offer valuable insights, further research with rigorous control of confounding variables is necessary to determine whether these relationships are causal.

2.3 Neck-related shoulder pain neurophysiology

To provide a rationale for shoulder pain produced or influenced by the cervical spine, it is needed to understand referred pain mechanisms.

Pain originating from the cervical spine can extend beyond the neck, affecting the shoulder, upper limb, and even the anterior or posterior chest wall. Structures such as zygapophyseal joints (**Figure 1**), ligaments, muscles, and intervertebral discs have been identified as potential sources of this referred pain. Studies have demonstrated that stimulating lower cervical spine joint levels (C4-T1) can trigger pain in the shoulder and upper limb [55–59], supporting the idea that cervical dysfunction may contribute to symptoms in these areas. Similarly, mechanical and electrical stimulation of intervertebral discs has been associated with pain in the posterior thorax and scapular region, further reinforcing the cervical spine's role in referred pain [60].

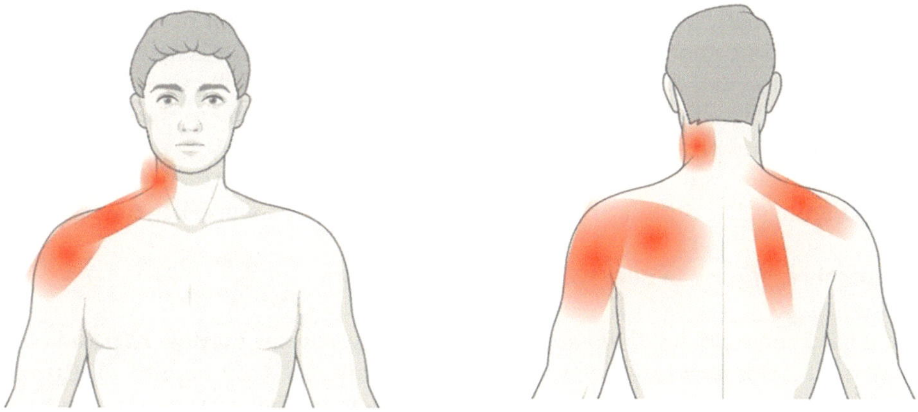

Figure 1.
Shoulder referred pain from C5–C6 and C6–C7 cervical facet joints. Adapted from Cooper et al. [55]. Edited by biorender.com

Interestingly, evidence suggests that neck-related shoulder pain can sometimes be alleviated through interventions targeting the shoulder itself. In one study, 30 out of 34 patients experienced neck pain relief following lidocaine and cortisone infiltration in the subacromial space, thus underscoring the complex relationship between cervical and shoulder pain [61].

Although patterns of referred pain from cervical structures have been documented, pinpointing the exact structure responsible for generating symptoms remains challenging [62]. This difficulty aligns with the understanding that pain is not merely a direct response to tissue damage but rather an inferential process that integrates multisensory information [63]. Consequently, even if a therapy successfully alleviates symptoms, this does not necessarily confirm the treated area as the origin of the pain.

These considerations are essential when interpreting pain through biopsychosocial and enactive models, which emphasize its complexity and the interplay of biological, psychological, and social factors [5, 64–66]. Therefore, a comprehensive approach to pain assessment and treatment should account for these multidimensional influences rather than focusing solely on anatomical sources.

Even if the exact mechanisms of referred cervical pain remain unclear, some studies suggest that the convergence of afferent pathways in the central nervous system may play a crucial role. This convergence implies that the central nervous system receives afferent fibers from two different peripheral areas through the same second-order neuron, which carries the information to the brain. Because of this, an afference from one of the zones can be interpreted as coming from the other [67].

In the case of referred cervical pain, afferences from the cervical spine converge with neurons that carry afferences from peripheral regions such as the chest wall, upper limb, or head, which may explain referred pain in the shoulder from the cervical spine [60]. Despite being able to explain part of the underlying mechanisms of this phenomenon, the convergence theory seems insufficient due to various intrinsic aspects of referred pain: it depends on the intensity of nociception, appears with a temporal delay from the onset of nociception, and often is extrasegmental. In this regard, referred pain largely depends on neuroplastic changes that might be associated with central sensitization [68]. Among these changes lies the genesis of new collateral synapses in the dorsal horn of the spinal cord in different spinal segments. In other words, if nociceptive stimulation is intense or persistent (intensity and duration of the stimulus), the overstimulation of dorsal horn neurons predisposes them to generate action potentials that promote the development of this new network of collateral synapses at different levels of the spinal cord. This will cause the expansion of medullar receptive fields, different from those corresponding to the initial damaged area (wind-up phenomenon). For this reason, patients may develop symptoms in distant areas different from the injured zone, even in extrasegmental areas, this being something that could not be fully explained by the convergence theory.

2.4 Clinical reasoning in neck-related shoulder pain

As it has been reported that shoulder and neck symptoms may overlap and confuse clinicians [28], it is necessary to guide physical evaluation within a clinical reasoning framework. In that context, clinical history data may predispose the therapist to carry out a cervical assessment in a shoulder pain patient. For instance, neck pain coexisting with shoulder symptoms [55], experiencing neck pain prior to the shoulder's symptoms onset [34], a diagnosis of rotator cuff-related shoulder pain [20], a decrease of cervical range of motion [62, 69], shoulder symptoms modification with neck movements [62], non-clear shoulder pain diagnosis, conserved shoulder range of motion [27, 62], previous cervical surgery [70, 71], bilateral symptoms or symptoms distal to the elbow might be some examples. Finally, the presence of centralization after neck treatment has been reported to be associated with cervical contribution [34].

3. Treating the neck in shoulder pain patients

3.1 Repeated movements

Neck-related shoulder pain patients have been largely considered from the MDT system [72], with several research published in this matter, including case reports [8, 73], case studies [22, 23], and observational studies [24, 26, 74].

In the observational studies, shoulder patients improved their symptoms with neck repeated movements, thus considering them 'Cervical Derangement' patients, that is, neck-related shoulder patients. That happened in 29% of subjects (n = 82), with a full resolution of symptoms in 37% after 2 weeks and in 82% of them after 4 weeks [24]. Similarly, it was reported in 47.6% of 84 subjects [74] and in 17% of 316 participants [26]. Finally, the highest prevalence data of cervical contribution has been reported at 50% in a 60 subjects' sample, with this consideration not being exclusively related to the MDT system [34].

3.2 Spinal mobilizations with arm movements

From a similar perspective, the Mulligan Concept also proposes some approaches to address shoulder pain with cervical treatment: under its Spinal Mobilization With Arm Movements (SMWAM), it employs passive accessory cervical mobilization associated with active shoulder movement to improve restricted or painful shoulder movements [75]. Related to this, the importance of mobilizing the C4 vertebra has been reported, as it allows stimulation of the cervical nerve C5, responsible for a significant portion of shoulder innervation [76].

3.3 Passive accessory mobilizations

Similarly, it has been demonstrated that classical joint mobilization techniques, such as posterior-anterior and anterior-posterior mobilizations, lateral glides, and cervical manipulations, may improve shoulder pain and function [77–83], showing similar effects regardless of the different applied mobilization modalities [77]. Furthermore, cervical mobilizations seem to induce hypoalgesia and sympathoexcitatory effects, which could be reached by the activation of the descending inhibitory mechanisms of the periaqueductal gray matter, as well as induce changes in cervical muscle function [84].

To the best of the author's knowledge, there is only one study that has demonstrated the lack of value of cervical treatment in shoulder pathology, as no benefit was found in adding cervical manual therapy to the impingement treatment [85]. Considering the discrepancy with other research, the authors themselves propose possible justifications such as the lack of dosage in the administered treatment or the potential ineffectiveness of treating the cervical spine in patients without concomitant cervical problems [85].

4. Conclusions

The shoulder region and cervical spine may work as an inseparable functional pair due to their neurophysiological, metameric, biomechanical, and myofascial connections. While lower back origin is commonly considered for gluteal, groin, or leg pain, cervical influence is not commonly taken into account for shoulder patients. Similarly, the lack of defined and standardized evaluation tools and diagnostic labeling is a major limitation that might severely impact the decision-making and clinical reasoning processes in clinical practice, as well as the homogeneity of selection criteria applied to different samples in research.

Repeated cervical movements improving shoulder symptoms, cervical mobility reproducing or modifying shoulder symptoms, or radicular symptoms are factors typically described to identify cervical involvement in SP. However, there is no standardized criteria or studies verifying the reliability of these examinations. Most studies only consider cervical involvement in cases of radicular pain or radiculopathy, but do not encompass the idea of the cervical spine as a participant in potential somatic shoulder referred pain.

This reality might lead to unintentionally heterogeneous samples in research. Shoulder pain patients with CC might be included in studies investigating treatment effectiveness for other specific shoulder pathologies. Therefore, overlooking this clinical diagnosis may result in misguided or misdirected treatments: directing treatment to the shoulder in a patient with cervical involvement compromises treatment effects and makes research and clinical applicability imprecise [35].

The exposed data underline the need for further research to enhance the understanding of this clinical phenomenon. While cervical involvement is gaining attention in literature, it remains one of the commonly overlooked hypotheses when diagnosing shoulder patients. Despite this, what seems to be clear is that the cervical spine should be examined before attempting any specific shoulder diagnosis [28]. Although its high prevalence has been reported, a proposal on how to diagnose this condition still needs to be established.

Acknowledgements

We acknowledge Universidad Francisco de Vitoria for allowing this publication with the funding UFV2025-35.

Conflict of interest

The authors declare no conflict of interest.

Author details

Alberto Roldán-Ruiz* and Gabriele Bertotti
School of Physiotherapy, Faculty of Health Sciences, Universidad Francisco de Vitoria, Madrid, Spain

*Address all correspondence to: alberto.roldan@ufv.es

References

[1] Hind J, GAS S, Arealis G, Khadabadi N, Ashwood N. An algorithmic approach to shoulder pathology. Journal of Family Medicine and Primary Care. 2022;**11**:5510

[2] House J, Mooradian A. Evaluation and management of shoulder pain in primary care clinics. Southern Medical Journal. 2010;**103**:1129-1137. Available from: http://www.ncbi.nlm.nih.gov/pubmed/20890250

[3] Mitchell C, Adebajo A, Hay E, Carr A. Shoulder pain: Diagnosis and management in primary care. BMJ. 2005;**331**:1124-1128. Available from: http://www.ncbi.nlm.nih.gov/pubmed/16282408

[4] May S, Chance-Larsen K, Littlewood C, Lomas D, Saad M. Reliability of physical examination tests used in the assessment of patients with shoulder problems: A systematic review. Physiotherapy. 2010;**96**:179-190. DOI: 10.1016/j.physio.2009.12.002

[5] Gifford L. Pain, the tissues and the nervous system: A conceptual model. Physiotherapy. 1998;**84**:27-36. Available from: http://linkinghub.elsevier.com/retrieve/pii/S0031940605659007

[6] Arendt-Nielsen L, Fernández-de-las-Peñas C, Graven-Nielsen T. Basic aspects of musculoskeletal pain: From acute to chronic pain. Journal of Manual & Manipulative Therapy. 2011;**19**:186-193. Available from: http://www.tandfonline.com/doi/full/10.1179/106698111X13129729551903

[7] Sergienko S, Kalichman L. Myofascial origin of shoulder pain: A literature review. Journal of Bodywork and Movement Therapies. 2015;**19**:91-101. Available from: http://www.ncbi.nlm.nih.gov/pubmed/25603748

[8] Menon A, May S. Shoulder pain: Differential diagnosis with mechanical diagnosis and therapy extremity assessment – A case report. Manual Therapy. 2013;**18**:354-357. Available from: http://www.ncbi.nlm.nih.gov/pubmed/22795390

[9] Borstad J, Woeste C. The role of sensitization in musculoskeletal shoulder pain. Brazilian Journal of Physical Therapy. 2015;**19**:251-257. Available from: http://www.ncbi.nlm.nih.gov/pubmed/26443971

[10] Fillingim RB. Individual differences in pain: Understanding the mosaic that makes pain personal. Pain. 2017;**158**:S11-S18

[11] Mallick-Searle T, Sharma K, Toal P, Gutman A. Pain and function in chronic musculoskeletal pain—Treating the whole person. Journal of Multidisciplinary Healthcare. 2021;**14**:335-347

[12] Schibany N, Zehetgruber H, Kainberger F, Wurnig C, Ba-Ssalamah A, Herneth AM, et al. Rotator cuff tears in asymptomatic individuals: A clinical and ultrasonographic screening study. European Journal of Radiology. 2004;**51**:263-268. Available from: http://www.ncbi.nlm.nih.gov/pubmed/15294335

[13] Bradley MP, Tung G, Green A. Overutilization of shoulder magnetic resonance imaging as a diagnostic screening tool in patients with chronic shoulder pain. Journal of Shoulder and Elbow Surgery. 2005;**14**:233-237

[14] Schellingerhout JM, Verhagen AP, Thomas S, Koes BW. Lack of uniformity in diagnostic labeling of shoulder pain: Time for a different approach. Manual Therapy. 2008;**13**:478-483. Available from: http://www.ncbi.nlm.nih.gov/pubmed/18555732

[15] de Winter AF, Jans MP, Scholten RJ, Devillé W, van Schaardenburg D, Bouter LM. Diagnostic classification of shoulder disorders: Interobserver agreement and determinants of disagreement. Annals of the Rheumatic Diseases. 1999;**58**:272-277. Available from: http://www.ncbi.nlm.nih.gov/pubmed/10225810

[16] Carter T, Hall H, McIntosh G, Murphy J, MacDougall J, Boyle C. Intertester reliability of a classification system for shoulder pain. Physiotherapy. 2012;**98**:40-46. Available from: http://www.ncbi.nlm.nih.gov/pubmed/22265384

[17] Juel NG, Natvig B. Shoulder diagnoses in secondary care, a one year cohort. BMC Musculoskeletal Disorders. 2014;**15**:89. Available from: http://bmcmusculoskeletdisord.biomedcentral.com/articles/10.1186/1471-2474-15-89

[18] Storheil B, Klouman E, Holmvik S, Emaus N, Fleten N. Intertester reliability of shoulder complaints diagnoses in primary health care. Scandinavian Journal of Primary Health Care. 2016;**34**:224-231. Available from: http://www.ncbi.nlm.nih.gov/pubmed/27404451

[19] Artus M, Holt TA, Rees J. The painful shoulder: An update on assessment, treatment, and referral. The British Journal of General Practice. 2014;**64**:e593-e595. Available from: http://www.ncbi.nlm.nih.gov/pubmed/25179075

[20] Roldán-Ruiz A, Bailón-Cerezo J, Torres-Lacomba M. The prevalence of subclassification-based diagnoses when considering cervical contribution in shoulder pain patients: A secondary analysis from a previous research. Journal of Manual & Manipulative Therapy. 2024:1-9 [Online ahead of print]

[21] ÖstÖr AJK, Richards CA, Prevost AT, Speed CA, Hazleman BL. Diagnosis and relation to general health of shoulder disorders presenting to primary care. Rheumatology. 2005;**44**:800-805

[22] Hathcock JA, Boyer CW, Morris JB. Shoulder pain of spinal source in the military: A case series. Military Medicine. 2022;**187**:e1240-e1246

[23] Pheasant S. Cervical contribution to functional shoulder impingement: Two case reports. International Journal of Sports Physical Therapy. 2016;**11**:980-991. Available from: http://www.ncbi.nlm.nih.gov/pubmed/27904800%0Ahttp://www.pubmedcentral.nih.gov/articlerender.fcgi?artid=PMC5095950

[24] Heidar Abady A, Rosedale R, Chesworth BM, Rotondi MA, Overend TJ. Application of the McKenzie system of Mechanical Diagnosis and Therapy (MDT) in patients with shoulder pain; a prospective longitudinal study. Journal of Manual & Manipulative Therapy. 2017;**9817**:1-9. Available from: https://www.tandfonline.com/doi/full/10.1080/10669817.2017.1313929

[25] Rosedale R, Rastogi R, Kidd J, Lynch G, Supp G, Robbins SM. A study exploring the prevalence of Extremity Pain of Spinal Source (EXPOSS). Journal of Manual & Manipulative Therapy. 2019;**28**(4):222-230. Available from: https://www.tandfonline.com/doi/full/10.1080/10669817.2019.1661706

[26] Karel YHJM, Scholten-Peeters GGM, Thoomes-de Graaf M, Duijn E, van Broekhoven JB, Koes BW, et al. Physiotherapy for patients with shoulder pain in primary care: A descriptive study of diagnostic- and therapeutic management. Physiotherapy. 2017;**103**:369-378

[27] Maccio JR, Carlton L, Levesque K, Maccio JG, Egan L. Directional preference of the extremity: A preliminary investigation. Journal of Manual & Manipulative Therapy. 2018;**26**:272-280

[28] Katsuura Y, Bruce J, Taylor S, Gullota L, Kim HJ. Overlapping, masquerading, and causative cervical spine and shoulder pathology: A systematic review. Global Spine Journal. 2020;**10**:195-208

[29] Kulkarni R, Gibson J, Brownson P, Thomas M, Rangan A, Carr AJ, et al. Subacromial shoulder pain. Shoulder Elbow. 2015;7:135-143

[30] Holmes RE, Barfield WR, Woolf SK. Clinical evaluation of nonarthritic shoulder pain: Diagnosis and treatment. The Physician and Sportsmedicine. 2015;**43**:262-268

[31] Bokshan SL, DePasse JM, Eltorai AEM, Paxton ES, Green A, Daniels AH. An evidence-based approach to differentiating the cause of shoulder and cervical spine pain. The American Journal of Medicine. 2016;**129**:913-918. Available from: http://www.ncbi.nlm.nih.gov/pubmed/27155111

[32] Thomas Quin Throckmorton PKJEKRCS. Differentiating cervical spine and shoulder pathology: Common disorders and key points of evaluation and treatment. Instructional Course Lectures. 2014;**63**:401-408

[33] Requejo-Salinas N, Fernández-Matías R, Cadogan A, Chester R, Roy J-S, Struyf F, et al. Neck or shoulder? Establishing consensus for spine screening in patients with shoulder pain: An international modified Delphi study. Physical Therapy. 2024;**105**(2):pzae133

[34] Roldán-Ruiz A, Bailón-Cerezo J, Falla D, Torres-Lacomba M. The prevalence of cervical contribution in patients reporting shoulder pain. An observational study. Musculoskeletal Science & Practice. 2024;**73**:103158

[35] Walker T, Salt E, Lynch G, Littlewood C. Screening of the cervical spine in subacromial shoulder pain: A systematic review. Shoulder Elbow. 2018;**11**(4):305-315. Available from: http://journals.sagepub.com/doi/10.1177/1758573218798023

[36] Walker T, Cuff A, Salt E, Lynch G, Littlewood C. Examination of the neck when a patient complains of shoulder pain: A global survey of current practice (2019). Musculoskeletal Care. 2020;**18**:256-264

[37] Laslett M. Evidence-based diagnosis and treatment of the painful sacroiliac joint. The Journal of Manual & Manipulative Therapy. 2008;**16**:142-152. Available from: http://www.ncbi.nlm.nih.gov/pubmed/19119403

[38] Heidar Abady A, Rosedale R, Chesworth BM, Rotondi MA, Overend TJ. Consistency of commonly used orthopedic special tests of the shoulder when used with the McKenzie system of mechanical diagnosis and therapy. Musculoskeletal Science & Practice. 2018;**33**:11-17. Available from: http://www.ncbi.nlm.nih.gov/pubmed/29059632

[39] Cannon DE, Dillingham TR, Miao H, Andary MT, Pezzin LE. Musculoskeletal

disorders in referrals for suspected cervical radiculopathy. Archives of Physical Medicine and Rehabilitation. 2007;**88**:1256-1259

[40] Roberson TA, Jew NB, Azar FM, Mauck BM, Dockery JD, Throckmorton TW. Cervical radiculitis presenting as shoulder pain. Current Orthopaedic Practice. 2015;**26**:521-525

[41] Rebelatto MN, Alburquerque-Sendín F, Gava V, Camargo PR, Haik MN. Cervical sensitivity, range of motion and strength in individuals with shoulder pain: A cross-sectional case control study. Musculoskeletal Science & Practice. 2023;**67**:102834

[42] Fonseca Fialho HR, Gava V, Fonseca RNS, Kamonseki DH, Barbosa GM. Thinking outside the shoulder: A systematic review and metanalysis of kinetic chain characteristics in non-athletes with shoulder pain. PLoS One. 2024;**19**:e0314909

[43] Takasaki H, Hall T, Kaneko S, Iizawa T, Ikemoto Y. Cervical segmental motion induced by shoulder abduction assessed by magnetic resonance imaging. Spine (Phila Pa 1976). 2009;**34**:E122-E126. Available from: http://www.ncbi.nlm.nih.gov/pubmed/19179912

[44] Theodoridis D, Ruston S. The effect of shoulder movements on thoracic spine 3D motion. Clinical Biomechanics. 2002;**17**:418-421

[45] Meurer A, Grober J, Betz U, Decking J, Rompe J-D. Die BWS-Beweglichkeit von Impingementpatienten im Vergleich zu Gesunden - eine inklinometrische Studie. Zeitschrift für Orthopädie und Ihre Grenzgebiete. 2004;**142**:415-420

[46] Theisen C, van Wagensveld A, Timmesfeld N, Efe T, Heyse TJ, Fuchs-Winkelmann S, et al. Co-occurrence of outlet impingement syndrome of the shoulder and restricted range of motion in the thoracic spine - A prospective study with ultrasound-based motion analysis. BMC Musculoskeletal Disorders. 2010;**11**:135

[47] Hunter DJ, Rivett DA, McKeirnan S, Smith L, Snodgrass SJ. Relationship between shoulder impingement syndrome and thoracic posture. Physical Therapy. 2020;**100**:677-686

[48] Manoso-Hernando D, Bailón-Cerezo J, Elizagaray-García I, Achútegui-García-Matres P, Suárez-Díez G, Gil-Martínez A. Cervical and thoracic spine mobility in rotator cuff related shoulder pain: A comparative analysis with asymptomatic controls. Journal of Functional Morphology and Kinesiology. 2024;**9**:128

[49] Falla D, Jull G, Hodges PW. Feedforward activity of the cervical flexor muscles during voluntary arm movements is delayed in chronic neck pain. Experimental Brain Research. 2004;**157**:43-48. Available from: http://www.ncbi.nlm.nih.gov/pubmed/14762639

[50] Falla D, Rainoldi A, Merletti R, Jull G. Spatio-temporal evaluation of neck muscle activation during postural perturbations in healthy subjects. Journal of Electromyography and Kinesiology. 2004;**14**:463-474. Available from: http://www.ncbi.nlm.nih.gov/pubmed/15165596

[51] Gurfinkel VS, Lipshits MI, Lestienne FG. Anticipatory neck muscle activity associated with rapid arm movements. Neuroscience Letters. 1988;**94**:104-108. Available from: http://www.ncbi.nlm.nih.gov/pubmed/3241659

[52] Asker M, Ravnanger J, Bjørnstad T, Skillgate E. Correlation between neck motor control impairment and shoulder pain in elite male handball players. Journal of Science and Medicine in Sport. 2014;**18**:e76. Available from: https://linkinghub.elsevier.com/retrieve/pii/S144024401400526X

[53] Wannaprom N, Treleaven J, Jull G, Uthaikhup S. Response rate and comparison of clinical features associated with positive or negative responses to a scapular positioning test in patients with neck pain and altered scapular alignment: A cross-sectional study. BMJ Open. 2021;**11**:e057459

[54] Takasaki H, Herbowy S. Immediate improvement in the cranio-cervical flexion test associated with MDT-based interventions: A case report. Journal of Manual & Manipulative Therapy. 2016;**24**:285-292

[55] Cooper G, Bailey B, Bogduk N. Cervical zygapophysial joint pain maps. Pain Medicine. 2007;**8**:344-353

[56] Dwyer A, Aprill C, Bogduk N. Cervical zygapophyseal joint pain patterns. I: A study in normal volunteers. Spine (Phila Pa 1976). 1990;**15**:453-457. Available from: http://www.ncbi.nlm.nih.gov/pubmed/2402682

[57] Aprill C, Dwyer A, Bogduk N. Cervical zygapophyseal joint pain patterns. II: A clinical evaluation. Spine (Phila Pa 1976). 1990;**15**(6):458-461. Available from: http://www.ncbi.nlm.nih.gov/pubmed/2402683

[58] Schwarzer AC, Aprill CN, Derby R, Fortin J, Kine G, Bogduk N. The relative contributions of the disc and zygapophyseal joint in chronic low back pain. Spine (Phila Pa 1976). 1994;**19**:801-806. Available from: http://www.ncbi.nlm.nih.gov/pubmed/8202798

[59] Fukui S, Ohseto K, Shiotani M, Ohno K, Karasawa H, Naganuma Y, et al. Referred pain distribution of the cervical zygapophyseal joints and cervical dorsal rami. Pain. 1996;**68**:79-83. Available from: http://www.ncbi.nlm.nih.gov/pubmed/9252002

[60] Bogduk N. Innervation and pain patterns of the cervical spine. Physical Therapy of the Cervical and Thoracic Spine. 2002:61-72. DOI: 10.1016/B978-0-443-06564-4.50007-4. Available from: http://linkinghub.elsevier.com/retrieve/pii/B9780443065644500074

[61] Gorski JM, Schwartz LH. Shoulder impingement presenting as neck pain. The Journal of Bone and Joint Surgery-American Volume. 2003;**85**:635-638

[62] Rastogi R, Rosedale R, Kidd J, Lynch G, Supp G, Robbins SM. Exploring indicators of extremity pain of spinal source as identified by mechanical diagnosis and therapy (MDT): A secondary analysis of a prospective cohort study. Journal of Manual & Manipulative Therapy. 2022;**30**:172-179

[63] Tabor A, Thacker MA, Moseley GL, Körding KP. Pain: A statistical account. PLoS Computational Biology. 2017;**13**:e1005142

[64] Hadjistavropoulos T, Craig KD, Duck S, Cano A, Goubert L, Jackson PL, et al. A biopsychosocial formulation of pain communication. Psychological Bulletin. 2011;**137**:910-939. Available from: http://www.ncbi.nlm.nih.gov/pubmed/21639605

[65] Stilwell P, Harman K. An enactive approach to pain: Beyond the biopsychosocial model. Phenomenology and the Cognitive Sciences. 2019;**18**:637-665

[66] Gatchel RJ, Peng YB, Peters ML, Fuchs PN, Turk DC. The biopsychosocial

approach to chronic pain: Scientific advances and future directions. Psychological Bulletin. 2007;**133**:581-624. Available from: http://www.ncbi.nlm.nih.gov/pubmed/17592957

[67] Jin Q, Chang Y, Lu C, Chen L, Wang Y. Referred pain: Characteristics, possible mechanisms, and clinical management. Frontiers in Neurology. 2023;**14**:1104817

[68] Eadie M. James Ross (1837-1892) and his forgotten neurology textbook of 1881. Journal of the Royal College of Physicians of Edinburgh. 2010;**40**:263-268

[69] Norlander S, Aste-Norlander U, Nordgren B, Sahlstedt B. Mobility in the cervico-thoracic motion segment: An indicative factor of musculo-skeletal neck-shoulder pain. Scandinavian Journal of Rehabilitation Medicine. 1996;**28**:183-192. Available from: http://www.ncbi.nlm.nih.gov/pubmed/9122645

[70] Kholinne E, Kwak J, Sun Y, Lee H, Koh KH, Jeon I. Risk factors for persistent shoulder pain after cervical spine surgery. Orthopaedic Surgery. 2019;**11**:845-849

[71] Khan S, Hameed N, Mazar S, Hashmi IA, Rafi MS, Shah MI, et al. Persistent shoulder pain after anterior cervical discectomy and fusion (ACDF): Another dual pathology. Cureus. 2021;**13**(3):e13709

[72] McKenzie R. The Lumbar Spine : Mechanical Diagnosis and Therapy. Spinal Publications; 1981. ISBN 9780958364751

[73] Slaven EJ, Mathers J. Differential diagnosis of shoulder and cervical pain: A case report. Journal of Manual & Manipulative Therapy. 2010;**18**:191-196. Available from: http://www.ncbi.nlm.nih.gov/pubmed/22131792

[74] Rosedale R, Rastogi R, Kidd J, Lynch G, Supp G, Robbins SM. A study exploring the prevalence of Extremity Pain of Spinal Source (EXPOSS). Journal of Manual & Manipulative Therapy. 2020;**28**:222-230

[75] Mulligan BR. Spinal Mobilization with Arm Movement. Adapted by Manual Therapy "NAGs", "SNAGs", "MWMs", Etc. 6th ed. Plane View Services; 2006. ISBN 101877520039

[76] Seo Y, Lee J, Han D. The effects of spinal mobilization with arm movements on shoulder muscle strengthening. Journal of Physical Therapy Science. 2015;**27**:11-13. Available from: http://www.ncbi.nlm.nih.gov/pubmed/25642026

[77] Hauswirth J, Ernst MJ, Preusser ML, Meichtry A, Kool J, Crawford RJ. Immediate effects of cervical unilateral anterior-posterior mobilisation on shoulder pain and impairment in post-operative arthroscopy patients. Journal of Back and Musculoskeletal Rehabilitation. 2017;**30**:615-623. Available from: http://www.ncbi.nlm.nih.gov/pubmed/28035910

[78] Wang SS, Meadows J. Immediate and carryover changes of C5-6 joint mobilization on shoulder external rotator muscle strength. Journal of Manipulative and Physiological Therapeutics. 2010;**33**:102-108. Available from: http://www.ncbi.nlm.nih.gov/pubmed/20170775

[79] Suter E, McMorland G. Decrease in elbow flexor inhibition after cervical spine manipulation in patients with chronic neck pain. Clinical Biomechanics (Bristol, Avon). 2002;**17**:541-544.

Available from: http://www.ncbi.nlm.nih.gov/pubmed/12206946

[80] Mintken PE, Cleland JA, Carpenter KJ, Bieniek ML, Keirns M, Whitman JM. Some factors predict successful short-term outcomes in individuals with shoulder pain receiving cervicothoracic manipulation: A single-arm trial. Physical Therapy. 2010;**90**:26-42. Available from: http://www.ncbi.nlm.nih.gov/pubmed/19959652

[81] McClatchie L, Laprade J, Martin S, Jaglal SB, Richardson D, Agur A. Mobilizations of the asymptomatic cervical spine can reduce signs of shoulder dysfunction in adults. Manual Therapy. 2009;**14**:369-374. Available from: http://www.ncbi.nlm.nih.gov/pubmed/18752983

[82] Bergman GJD, Winters JC, Groenier KH, Pool JJM, Jong BM, Postema K, et al. Manipulative therapy in addition to usual medical care for patients with shoulder dysfunction and pain. Annals of Internal Medicine. 2004;**141**:432. Available from: http://annals.org/article.aspx?doi=10.7326/0003-4819- 141-6-200409210-00008

[83] Schneider G. Restricted shoulder movement: Capsular contracture or cervical referral — A clinical study. The Australian Journal of Physiotherapy. 1989;**35**:97-100. Available from: http://www.ncbi.nlm.nih.gov/pubmed/25025266

[84] Sterling M, Jull G, Wright A. Cervical mobilisation: Concurrent effects on pain, sympathetic nervous system activity and motor activity. Manual Therapy. 2001;**6**:72-81. Available from: http://www.ncbi.nlm.nih.gov/pubmed/11414776

[85] Cook C, Learman K, Houghton S, Showalter C, O'Halloran B. The addition of cervical unilateral posterior-anterior mobilisation in the treatment of patients with shoulder impingement syndrome: A randomised clinical trial. Manual Therapy. 2014;**19**:18-24. DOI: 10.1016/j.math.2013.05.007

Section 2

Acute Traumatic Injuries

Chapter 3

Anterior Shoulder Dislocation

Svetoslav Dobrilov

Abstract

Anterior shoulder dislocation is the most common traumatic injury in the upper extremity. With increased sports activity among patients in different age groups, these injuries are becoming more frequent. First-time dislocators are becoming more important as a specific diagnosis and treatment group due to acquired pathology after shoulder dislocation. Improved diagnosis and evaluation of these pathological conditions in shoulder anatomy lead to appropriate treatment and fast and early recovery, especially in highly active athletes. Soft tissue injury (Bankart) and bony pathology (bone Bankart/Hill-Sachs) are still the most important issues that the surgeon had to diagnose properly, thus treat appropriately. Bony changes in shoulder anatomy are becoming more important, and a treatment algorithm should be specified.

Keywords: anterior shoulder dislocation, recurrent dislocation, glenoid bone loss, instability, humeral head bone loss

1. Introduction

The human shoulder is unique among the large joints in that it is the most mobile and used joint, even in the smallest routine movements. This range of motion is possible due to the interaction between the large humeral head and the small glenoid fossa. However, this is a prerequisite for instability and dislocation when reaching extreme ranges of motion. The stability of the joint is ensured by a delicate balance between static and dynamic stabilisers [1]. Static stabilisers are the glenoid labrum, glenohumeral ligaments, joint capsule, and rotator cuff. Dynamic stabilisers are the muscles around the scapula (rotator cuff) and the shoulder. Any imbalance in this relationship leads to instability of the joint and is a prerequisite for dislocation. Due to the fact that, in instability, the anatomical integrity is disrupted, especially of the static stabilisers, knowledge of their normal anatomy is essential.

Shoulder stability depends on the structural and functional relationship between these components. Of great importance for the functioning of the static stabilisers are the normal version of the glenoid and joint congruence, negative intra-articular pressure, the glenohumeral ligaments and the labrum. There is considerable variability in the "normal" version of the proximal humerus, according to Boileau and Walsh—a retroversion angle of approximately 20° compared to the transepicondylar axis of the distal humerus is characteristic of a large part of the population. Glenoid version is also variable relative to the axis of the scapula [2]. Despite the limiting and "stabilising" effect of the native retroversion of the bony anatomy of the glenohumeral joint, anterior dislocation, and instability remain the most common pathology. This chapter reviews the pathomorphological changes after anterior shoulder dislocation, the diagnostic options for their definition, and the therapeutic algorithm for treatment. Undoubtedly, this pathology brings with it shoulder instability, which, however, is not the main topic of this presentation, although the two topics are related.

2. Pathomorphology

Traumatic shoulder dislocation is a condition defined as a lack of contact between the articulating surfaces of the humeral head and the glenoid fossa. Of course, in the different types of shoulder dislocation, partial articular contact can be observed, but it is not sufficient to achieve movement.

The shoulder is the most commonly dislocated large joint [3, 4]. When the static and dynamic stabilisers are impaired, and the balance between movement and stability is disrupted, usually after an external force is applied, the result is glenohumeral/shoulder dislocation. The majority of dislocations occur in young patients between the ages of 20 and 30. Males predominate in about 85–90% of cases. The typical mechanism is trauma during physical activity or sports, when the arm is abducted to 90° and externally rotated. The subsequent external rotation and often extension causes a lever mechanism that dislocates the humeral head from the glenoid fossa. Another mechanism is a fall forward with the arm extended and adducted, although it is less common. Atraumatic dislocations occur mainly in multidirectional instability with predisposing factors such as hyperlaxity and are significantly less common.

The incidence of shoulder dislocations in the population is 1–2% or 8.3–12.3 per 100,000/year [5, 6]. There are several types of glenohumeral dislocation depending on the direction of dislocation of the humeral head relative to the glenoid fossa:

1. Anterior dislocation—the head of the humerus is anterior to the glenoid fossa and is subdivided into several subtypes:

    - *Subcoracoid*—the head is in front of the fossa but below the coracoid process.

    - *Subglenoid*—the humerus is anterior and inferior to the glenoid.

    - *Subclavicular*—the position of the head is anterior to the glenoid and medial to the coracoid process (inferior to the clavicle).

    - *Intrathoracic*—the head is anteromedial to the glenoid fossa, between the ribs.

2. Posterior dislocation—the head of the humerus lies behind the glenoid fossa. There are:

    - *Subacromial*—most common

    - *Subglenoid*—the head is located posteriorly and below the glenoid

    - *Subspinal*—medial to the acromion and below the scapular spine

3. Inferior dislocation (Luxatio erecta)—a rare injury in which the head of the humerus is located just below the glenoid fossa.

Over 95% of shoulder dislocations are anterior [7, 8]. The shoulder relies on static (bony and ligamentous structures and adhesion/cohesion) and dynamic (rotator cuff) stabilisers to maintain a stable position throughout the entire range of motion. During abduction and external rotation, the IGHL (inferior glenohumeral ligament) complex is the primary stabiliser against anterior glenohumeral translation.

In traumatic anterior humeral dislocation, the anteroinferior displacement of the humeral head stretches the capsuloligamentous structures, resulting in the disinsertion of the anteroinferior portion of the glenoid labrum (Bankart lesion). Other associated injuries may include Hill-Sachs lesions, SLAP lesions, capsular and rotator cuff tears, fractures of the glenoid rim (Bankart lesion), or the greater tubercle of the humerus.

The risk of recurrence after primary glenohumeral dislocation is highest in young patients, reaching 87% within the first 2 years, with rates even higher in athletes and physically active patients (86–100%) [9, 10]. This is due to acquired soft tissue and bone damage, early return to professional sports, and poor response to rehabilitation.

The incidence of recurrence after traumatic dislocation among young patients is significantly higher and reaches 66–94% under 20 years of age, 92% in patients aged 14–17 years, and 50–64% under 30 years of age [11–13].

2.1 Soft tissue pathomorphology

There are several pathological changes associated with the anteroinferior aspect of the glenoid labrum. A Bankart lesion is classically described as a disinsertion/detachment of the anteroinferior labrum along with the entrapped inferior glenohumeral complex (IGHL). Bankart initially described the disinsertion of the labrum in four patients with glenohumeral instability and referred to it as an "essential lesion." He later reported excellent results after labral reattachment (Bankart procedure) in 27 patients. A Bankart lesion occurs in 93.7% of chronic instability cases and in 78.2% of acute instability cases. Sugaya et al., in a study of 100 patients, found a Bankart lesion in 97 of them [14]. Similar data have been reported by many other authors [15, 16].

Shields et al., in a study of patients with anterior shoulder dislocation, found that 87% of cases had labral damage, and 79% had anterior capsule insufficiency [8]. Baker et al., in an arthroscopic study of traumatic dislocations, found 13% capsular damage, 25% partial disinsertion (moderate Bankart) and 62% combined damage [17]. Larrain et al., in a study of patients with traumatic instability, found capsular damage in only 4%, partial labral disinsertion in 32%, and capsular tear and Bankart damage in 64% [18].

Neviaser described the so-called ALPSA lesion (anterior labral periosteal sleeve avulsion), which closely resembles a Bankart lesion but with one important difference: the anterior scapular periosteum is not torn, and the inferior glenohumeral ligament, labrum, and periosteum are "slipped" and displaced like a sleeve, medial to the glenoid neck [19].

Open treatment of glenohumeral instability has a high success rate, and although arthroscopic Bankart refixation is currently preferred because of its atraumatic nature, it does not always have consistently reliable results. The rate of poor and unsatisfactory results ranges from 5% to 60% [20, 21].

Glenoid labral tear (GLAD) is a lesion first described by Neviaser as an articular lesion of the anterior inferior glenoid in combination with labral damage [22]. These lesions are rare and occur predominantly in young patients under 20 years of age who are actively involved in sports. However, they are challenging due to the complex chondral and labral damage.

The SLAP lesions described by Snyder et al. were not initially considered to be a consequence of shoulder dislocation [23]. Later, in a group of patients with glenohumeral instability, anteroinferior labral and SLAP lesions were found [24]. All shoulders had a complex labral disinsertion from 10′ o'clock to 6′ o'clock (in right shoulders) of the glenoid, corresponding to the entire posterosuperior, anterosuperior, and anteroinferior labrum. Snyder et al. defined several types of SLAP lesions: type I (11%) is a separation of the edge of the superior labrum; type II (41%) is an avulsion of the labral-bicipital complex from the glenoid; type III (33%) a displaced bucket-handle tear with intact biceps tendon insertion and type IV (15%) is a dislocated type III tear but with involvement of the biceps tendon fibres [23]. Maffet et al. added three more types to this classification [25]. Athletes using repetitive overhead arm movements are prone to types I and II, while types III, IV, or VI are more typical of falls on an outstretched arm. Types V and VII are characteristic of patients with chronic instability [26].

Capsular avulsion from the humerus following shoulder dislocation was first described by Nicola, and later, the lesion was defined in detail by Wolf as humeral avulsion of the anterior glenohumeral ligament (HAGL) [27]. This term is used to refer to lesions of the anterior glenohumeral ligament. Later, the term reverse HAGL (RHAGL/PHAGL) came into use for lesions of the humeral insertion of the posterior inferior glenohumeral ligament. In 2007, Bui-Mansfield classified six types of HAGL lesions. They occur in about 7–10% of arthroscopic operations and in 1–10% of patients with glenohumeral instability [28].

Rotator cuff tear in young patients is usually partial-thickness on the articular side. This is the result of eccentric loading of the tendon during recurrent instability. A full-thickness tear occurs in patients over 40 years of age and is suspected if there is no motion and persistent pain 3 weeks after the primary dislocation [29].

There are multiple anatomical factors related to the stability of the glenohumeral joint. Joint congruence has a concave-compression effect, which could be altered due to glenoid dysplasia or fracture. The function of the glenoid labrum is to increase the depth of the fossa and articular surface and to provide additional stability. Around it, there are multiple ligament attachments. After the Bankart lesion, detachment of the capsule or ligaments leads to instability. Negative intra-articular pressure has a vacuum effect on the joint. Glenohumeral ligaments are restrictors to a certain range of motion, and their damage is responsible for a great number of instability cases. Other minor stabilisers are the posterior capsule and rotator cuff. Long head of the biceps tendon is a dynamic limiter of the anterior and superior translation of the humeral head, and SLAP tears could lead to motion-related shoulder pain.

In addition to soft tissue pathoanatomical changes, glenohumeral instability also involves bony changes—of the humeral head, the glenoid labrum, or both. When bony changes contribute to the instability, it can be defined as "complex." The importance of bony defects increases gradually after multiple recurrences of instability, after a soft tissue stabilisation procedure.

2.2 Bone pathomorphology

Current understanding of the pathomorphology of anterior shoulder dislocation defines bony defects of the glenoid and humeral head as almost mandatory [11, 30–34]. They lead to instability because they alter the morphology of the articulating surfaces and the surrounding stabilising factors [35].

Several studies have demonstrated extremely unsatisfactory results after isolated soft tissue stabilisation without taking into account significant bony changes in the glenoid articular facet [11, 30–34]. Their high incidence in first-time dislocators is the main reason for this [36–38].

Greis et al. [39] presented the effect of progressive labral and bone loss of the articulating surfaces and the change in pressure of the glenohumeral joint under compressive loading. Reduction of the amount of labral tissue in the anteroinferior part decreases the contact area by 7–15% compared to intact shoulders and increases the contact pressure by 8–20%. With bone loss corresponding to 30% of the glenoid diameter, the contact area of the entire glenoid decreases by 41%, and the contact pressure of the entire glenoid increases by 100%, while in the anteroinferior quadrant, it is between 300% and 400%. Because of the progressive bone wear in this area, as well as the increased pressure, a soft tissue (Bankart) stabilisation procedure subjects the soft tissues to the above-mentioned loads. This inevitably leads to a compromise of the procedure.

Traumatic shoulder dislocation is associated with a bony defect in the glenoid and can lead to glenohumeral instability in a high percentage of cases. The literature reports an 80–90% incidence in patients with chronic posttraumatic glenohumeral instability [14, 34]. Instability increases proportionally with defect size, and larger defects have a worse prognosis after soft tissue stabilisation [40, 41].

In the acute period after glenohumeral dislocation (within 3 months), fracture fragments of the anterior glenoid may be present. As instability becomes chronic (>6 months), partial resorption of the fragments begins [42]. More than half of patients with chronic instability do not have a clearly identifiable bone fragment. With the recurrence of instability, the bone defects may become more extensive (**Figure 1**).

Approximately 70% of patients with a primary dislocation are at risk for recurrence within the next 2 years, although this is highly dependent on age. In patients under 20 years of age, the risk is 80%, in those 20–40 years of age, it is 60%, and it drops to 15% after the age of 40 [43, 44].

Edwards and Bigliani were among the first authors to grade the extent of bone loss, defining the term as erosive bone loss with a characteristic sclerotic and rounded contour of the inferior pole of the glenoid [32, 45]. In the early post-dislocation stage, approximately half of the patients have a clearly visible bone fragment, while in the remainder, it is difficult to visualise [32]. The clinical significance of these fragments nowadays is 13% of the glenoid width [46, 47].

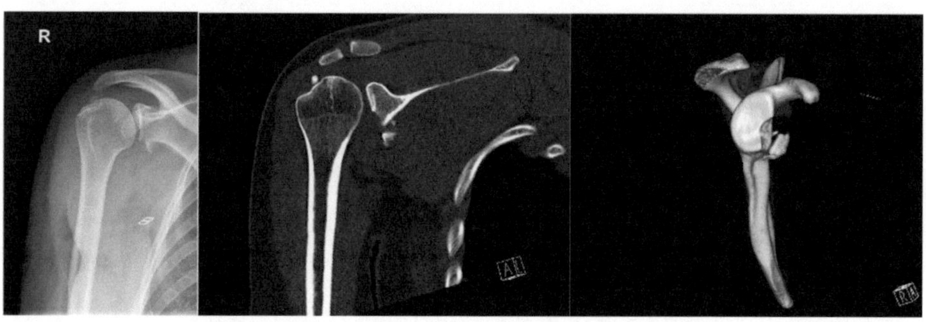

Figure 1.
Bony Bankart after first-time shoulder dislocation.

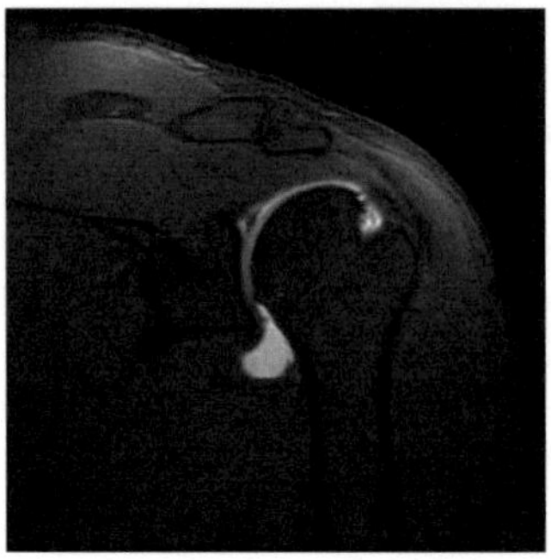

Figure 2.
Hill-Sachs defect.

The concept of "glenoid track" introduced by Itoi et al. [48] considers the interaction between glenoid and humeral bone loss resulting from shoulder dislocation. Therefore, a targeted search for a defect in the humeral head is of utmost importance (**Figure 2**).

In anterior shoulder dislocation, an impression fracture of the humeral head occurs in two-thirds of patients and increases with the frequency of recurrence [15]. In some studies, this rate reaches a worrying 95%, especially in magnetic resonance imaging (MRI) [7]. The calculation of the size of the defect is not always mandatory because of the interaction with the reciprocal glenoid defect. In other words, small humeral defects can lead to recurrence and vice versa—large defects can be clinically insignificant—the glenoid track concept.

Kaar et al. confirmed that, as the defect size increases, stability in abduction and external rotation decreases. Large defects of 5/8 of the radius of the humeral head reduce stability in this position. In defects of 7/8 of the radius, the defect leads to instability even in small abduction and neutral rotation [49].

Biomechanical studies by Sekiya et al. on cadavers concluded that isolated Hill-Sachs defects of 25% of the head volume caused significant translational instability of the humeral head [50]. Indications for treatment cannot be given solely on the size of the Hill-Sachs defect but rather on its position relative to the glenoid.

In modern terms, the relationship between the age of the patient at the time of the first dislocation and episodes of recurrent instability is indisputable [51]. The younger the patient (20 years as a cutoff), the higher the risk of recurrence, especially after soft tissue stabilisation in the presence of bone deficiency. Another important feature directly related to the above statement is the number of episodes of instability—with more than five episodes, the risk of instability increases by up to 40% [52]. Ultimately, the interaction of bipolar bone defects in risky shoulder positions—90° abduction and maximum external rotation is of greatest importance [40].

3. Diagnostics

3.1 Clinical diagnosis

The clinical diagnosis of a patient with anterior shoulder dislocation is not particularly difficult in the majority of cases. It may occur in overweight patients and neglected cases. However, it is essential to diagnose anterior shoulder instability, which is often the result of a single shoulder dislocation. Patients with glenoid loss report progressive relief of subluxation or complete dislocation in a given position. Although the assessment of instability is clear, attention should be paid to concomitant symptoms of rotator cuff damage (patients over 40 years), cartilage damage, SLAP lesions, etc.

The clinical examination includes a series of tests to assess anterior instability. The patient's shoulder girdle is inspected for abnormalities in position, pigmentation, muscle wasting/atrophy, scarring, and deformities. Range of motion is assessed actively and passively, including flexion-extension, adduction-abduction, and rotation, the latter being assessed at 0° and 90° adduction. Due to the fact that GH instability is defined as a condition in which the humeral head cannot remain centred in the glenoid fossa, it is important for the patient to demonstrate (if possible) their functional problem.

Provocative (stress) tests examine the ability of the shoulder to resist forces that affect stability in positions where the ligaments are normally under tension. This occurs when the examiner places the patient's glenohumeral joint in a position that causes subluxation/luxation, pain, or discomfort. Most of these tests are performed while the patient is conscious, and the contralateral shoulder, which is considered "normal," is also tested.

3.1.1 Anterior apprehension test ("crank" test)

In this test, the patient is supine [53]. The examiner abducts the shoulder 90° and flexes the elbow at a right angle. With one hand, the humerus is slowly rotated externally, using the patient's forearm as a lever, while with the other hand, the humeral head is pushed forward. Under normal circumstances, no translation is observed because the anterior capsuloligamentous structures are intact. The test is considered positive when the patient feels that his shoulder is luxating and there is a deficit in the described structures.

The reverse manoeuvre is called the *relocation test*, where the examiner pushes the patient's humerus posteriorly, and the patient reports a sensation of displacement. This differentiates pain due to instability from pain due to other causes. In patients without instability, there is no change in sensation, whereas in those with instability, there is a decrease in pain. Many authors recommend performing *hyperlaxity tests* as part of the clinical examination [54]. Such an evaluation is recommended for patients with symptomatic traumatic instability and those with occult instability associated with pain. This is especially true in overhead sports [53].

3.2 Imaging diagnostics

See **Table 1**.

There is a wide variety of possible projections for assessing bone pathology (**Table 2**).

The specialised projection for comparing the glenoid width between the affected and healthy/contralateral side is the Bernageau projection. It provides sharp outlines in the form of a triangle, corresponding to the anterior inferior part of the glenoid. When the ratio of d1 of the affected glenoid to d2 of the healthy is $d1:d2 < 0.75$—the treatment recommendation is a coracoid transfer (Laterjet) (**Figure 3**) [54].

	Ultrasound	Radiography	MRI	Arthro-MRI	CT/+ contrast
Labral injury	++	–	++	++	–
Labral injury/SLAP	–	–	+/–	++	–
Bankart bone	++	+	+/–	++	++
Cartilage damage	–	–	+	+++	–
Glenoid geometry/fossa inclination	–	+	+++	+++	+++
Hill-Sachs defect	+++	+	+++	+++	+++
Rotator interval-biceps tendon and m. subscapularis	++	–	++	+++	–
Rotator cuff	+++	–	++	+++	–
Capsule engagement	+/–	–	+/–	++	–

Table 1.
Methods for imaging diagnosis of pathological findings in anterior shoulder instability.

Projection	Bone detail	Surrounding structures	Patient convenience	Hill-Sachs	Bankart bone
AP External rot. Internal rot.	+ +	+ +	+ +	– +	+/– +/–
Grashey	+/–	+/–	+	+/–	–
Garth	+/–	+/–	+	+	+
West point	+/–	+/–	–	+/–	+
Axillary	–	–	+/–	+/–	+
Scapular "Y"	–	–	+	–	–
Stryker notch	+/–	+/–	+/–	+	–
Bernageau view	+	+	+/–	+	+

Table 2.
Advantages and disadvantages of the projections used for instability diagnostics. (+) reliable; (+/–) indifferent; (–) unreliable.

3.2.1 Computer tomography (CT)

When we talk about anterior shoulder dislocation in a patient at risk for instability, it is advisable to perform a CT scan. Not infrequently, the patient's condition is painful, and he resists the various options for X-ray projection. CT also allows digital subtraction of the humerus, and thus, the glenoid can be analysed in more detail [11, 30]. Determining the degree of bone loss preoperatively helps to choose the right therapeutic approach. Other indications for this examination are recurrent dislocations; bilateral involvement, especially in the non-dominant hand; unsuccessful surgical procedure for stabilisation; dislocation after minimal trauma (primary) or minimal provocation; X-ray or MRI data of bone loss of the glenoid; instability

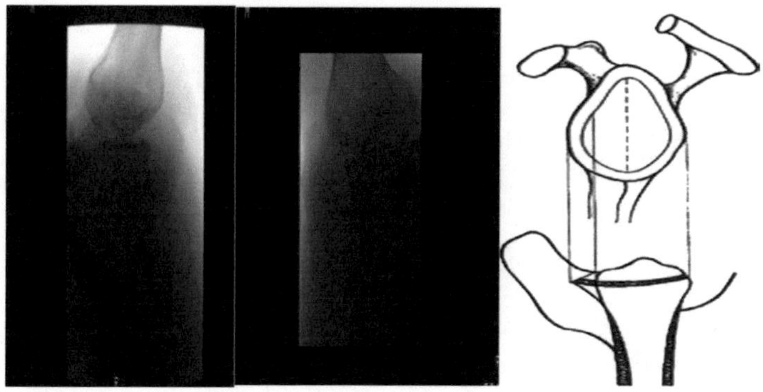

Figure 3.
Bernageau projection and the ratio of bone anatomy.

in the average volumes of movement. The existing CT methods for measuring the percentage of bone loss can be systematised in a table (**Table 3**) [55].

3.2.2 Magnetic resonance imaging (MRI)

This imaging sequence provides detailed information with respect to soft tissues. Of course, bony structures are also visible with a great amount of precision. The addition of intra-articular contrast enhances the delineation of anatomical features and increases the detection of hidden lesions associated with GH instability, particularly of the capsulolabral complex [56]. Simultaneous assessment of soft tissue damage and glenoid deficit in a single study has the undisputed advantage of reduced examination time and

Method of surfaces	(1) 3D CT image of the glenoid with humeral head subtraction. (2) An ideal circle is outlined in the lower 2/3 of the pyriform glenoid. (3) Bone loss is measured directly by the bone deficit within the circle.
Overlay method	(1) A perfect circle is drawn in the lower 2/3 of the pyriform glenoid of the affected and intact joint. (2) The circle on the unaffected side is digitally superimposed on the affected side. (3) Bone loss is calculated based on the difference in superimposition.
Pico/Pico methodology	(1) An ideal circle with the bare spot as its centre is drawn on the affected side using software, and the contact surface (A) is measured digitally. (2) After the overlay, the bone defect is also measured as a defect in the circle (D). (3) Bone loss is = D/A × 100%.
The front-to-back distance from the bearing point	(1) The load-bearing point is defined as the intersection of the transverse and longitudinal axes. (2) The distance from the load-bearing point to the anterior edge of the bone defect (A) and to the posterior edge (B) of the glenoid is defined. (3) Percentage bone loss = ([B 2 A]/2B) × 100%.
Measurement of Bankart bone	(1) A perfect circle with radius (R) is drawn in the lower 2/3 of the glenoid. (2) The length of the bone defect (x) is measured. (3) If x > R, the resistance to dislocation is >70% compared to an intact joint.
Ratio method	(1) A perfect circle with radius (R) is drawn in the lower 2/3 of the glenoid. (2) The distance from the centre of the circle to the anterior edge of the bone defect (d) is measured. (3) Bone loss is a percentage of the ratio d/R and a specialised mathematical function of (d) and (R).

Table 3.
Most important methods for quantification of bone loss after shoulder dislocation.

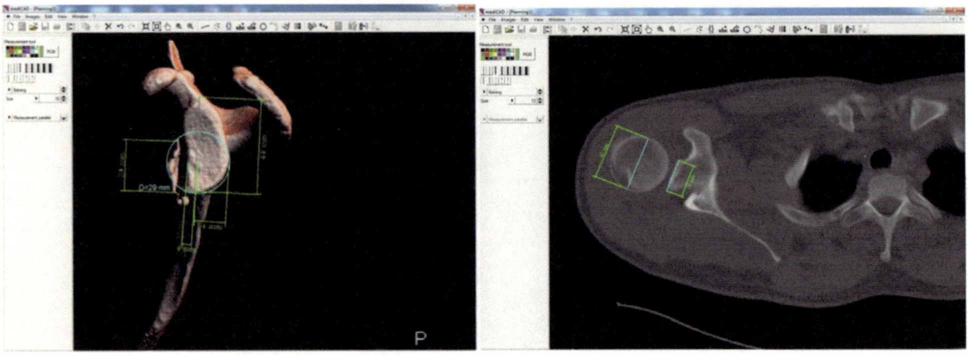

Figure 4.
Preoperative measurement of the degree of bone loss; AP/SI index (left) and TGHI (right).

cost. It also reduces the need for CT and the associated radiation exposure. Although 3D CT is the gold standard, MRI is increasingly being used to evaluate bony defects. The addition of contrast to it further increases its sensitivity, making it an extremely effective method for diagnosing capsulolabral pathology in shoulder instability [57].

3.3 Measuring the extent of bone loss

On a sagittal section, the glenoid joint face is selected (en face), and the longest (SI) and widest (AP) parts (diameter) of the glenoid fossa are determined; their intersection corresponds to the bare area. The ratio of the two values AP/SI is an index of the glenoid fossa with normal values around 0.7. A circle is drawn with the borders of the lower glenoid, and its radius (R) is determined. The length of the bone defect (x), if present, is determined, and the ratio between the two values is calculated from the data obtained when x > R, the resistance against dislocation is 70% of that of an intact joint.

In the same section, the lengths from the centre (bare spot) to the anterior (A) and posterior (B) glenoid rim were determined. Bone loss was determined using the formula (B – A)/2B × 100% defined by Sugaya [14]. The type of bone loss was again determined using Sugaya's criteria.

On an axial section, the ratio between the glenoid width at the bare spot level and the width of the humeral head is determined—transverse glenohumeral index (TGHI) (**Figure 4**). Its normal value is about 0.64. At values below 0.57, soft tissue stabilisation is at risk of recurrence and bone stabilisation is recommended. A specific element that we strictly apply is the *Instability Severity Index Score* (ISIS) score. This score allows for an assessment of the risk of recurrence of instability in high-risk patient groups. It is recommended to apply it both in acute dislocations and in chronic cases of recurrence. The algorithm we recommend is as follows: for ISIS <3, soft tissue stabilisation is recommended. For ISIS ≥ 3 but less than five dislocations, augmentation with free bone graft. ISIS ≥ 6 and chronic instability is an indication of coracoid transfer.

4. Treatment

Reduction of the dislocated shoulder in terms of emergency is out of discussion. Any delay leads to a risk of unstable reduction and/or neurovascular compromise [10]. The timeline for reduction is well established, but there are many reduction techniques in terms of the position of the patient, forces applied, position of the arm, etc. [58]. Those methods are highly dependent on the surgeon's preferences and experience, patient morphology and medical equipment. Local anaesthesia is widely used, but in muscular patients and those with neglected dislocations, it is not effective. Thus, sedation with propofol is the best treatment option, especially in cases with an inexperienced surgeon [59]. Closed reduction under local anaesthesia is successful in most acute dislocations. However, as long the shoulder stays dislocated, the reduction is more difficult, requires more force and increases the risk for additional iatrogenic damage. Reduction is also more complicated when facing muscular patients, uncooperative patients and those with suspected soft tissue interposition. Cases with glenoid fractures are not suitable for close reduction due to the risk of further damage.

Multiple studies evaluate optimal arm position, after reduction, for the management of anterior shoulder dislocation. The general consensus is to sling for 2 weeks in a neutral position. Some studies demonstrated a decreased risk of recurrence when immobilisation is in external rotation, compared to internal rotation/neutral position. Despite that, this is more uncomfortable for the patient [60]. The biomechanical explanation for this fact is that, in external rotation, the stress over the torn labrum is less [61]. Recent studies proved that, there were no major differences in terms of dislocation rate.

The duration of immobilisation in first-time dislocators is also a matter of debate. A significant reduction in the rate of recurrence has been stated in patients with immobilisation for 3 weeks compared to patients with immobilisation for 1 week (23% vs. 50%) [62]. Patients with prolonged duration of immobilisation (6 weeks) are showing improved functional outcomes compared to those with less long immobilisation (less than 6 weeks). However, there are some studies that prove the opposite. Paterson stated that, patients aged less than 30 years, who were kept in internal rotation for either less than 1 week or more than 3 weeks. The author found no significant differences in recurrence rate for patients in the first group compared with those who were immobilised for more than 3 weeks (41% vs. 37%) [63]. Although these controversies, immobilisation after anterior shoulder dislocation is obligatory in terms of patient comfort, especially in young, overhead/contact sports. An unexpected complication due to prolonged immobilisation and lack of early rehabilitation is shoulder stiffness and reduced ROM.

The general consensus in the literature is that young males who are practising contact sports are at significantly higher risk for recurrent instability than the general population. There is a strong correlation between sex and other risk factors, such as age or mechanism of injury, and young males are prone to instability events during contact sports [13]. A study by Robinson regarding recurrent instability for patients with no sports activity, noncontact sports and contact/overhead sports shows a high correlation between recurrence and overhead/contact sports- almost 14%; the other two groups have 62% and 43% recurrence rate [64].

Other authors demonstrate a high correlation between age and recurrence rate. Younger patients are more prone to redislocation in the first year, up to 50% under 20 years, and the percentage drops with age increase. This is related to the different biomechanical properties of collagen fibre type, capsule properties or changes in activity level as a function of age.

Surgical treatment in patients with first-time traumatic anterior shoulder dislocation depends on pathological findings. Major fracture fragments (glenoid fracture/greater tuberosity) had to be rigidly fixed when treating young, active overhead/contact sportsmen. Arthroscopic Bankart repair is the gold standard compared with open surgery and is recommended in patients younger than 30 years. Furthermore, arthroscopic stabilisation offers better shoulder mobility, satisfaction, and quicker return to activity time. Surgical repair is an appealing option for high-risk patients who have experienced traumatic anterior shoulder dislocation, are between the ages of 21 and 30 years, and participate in high-risk sports [13]. Recurrent instability after arthroscopic Bankart repair has been reported to be 8.1% and associated with younger patients, bilateral involvement, and closed reduction prior to repair [41]. Overall failure rates of Bankart repair, pooled from a meta-analysis of 12 studies, were found to be 13.7%. Higher rates of recurrence are expected in inexperienced surgeons, bad patient selection and overall improper diagnostic algorithms.

Larger bony deficits (≥20% from glenoid diameter) are not suitable for Bankart repair due to a higher risk of failure. In such cases, Laterjet (coracoid transfer) is the treatment recommendation [65]. This procedure has excellent long-term results, with reliable clinical outcomes and a low failure rate of 2–5% [66]. There are some considerations regarding early arthrosis and graft resorption. We observe great clinical results with this technique and minor radiological degenerative changes without clinical presentation. Regarding graft resorption, there are no instability episodes in the patient, even with more than 50% resorption of the graft.

The question about open or arthroscopic surgery is still an ongoing debate. Some studies present a higher recurrence of instability in arthroscopic treatment, but many surgeons advocate this with limitations in patient selection, technique used, etc. Overall, long-term clinical trials showed no significant difference in these two different algorithms [67]. A major systematic review focused on complications presents a higher complication rate in open techniques, compared to arthroscopic- 6.2% to 1.6%. Of course, these data should be commented on when comparing specific complications of both techniques, but not in general. In the end, it is all about correct clinical and imaging diagnosis, proper instability evaluation, and exact implication. When following these steps, excellent results are imminent.

5. Conclusion

Treating anterior shoulder dislocation is a complex procedure based on an established algorithm. Pathological changes during the first or multiple dislocations are important and dynamically connected. It is essential to be precise in diagnostics because this leads to appropriate treatment results. The most common findings are the Bankart lesion (incl. bony Bankart) and the Hill-Sachs lesion. Nevertheless, close reduction under anaesthesia and short immobilisation are standard approaches to this condition. More important are the next steps in order to evaluate pathology and correctly address it.

Younger and physically active patients under 25 years old are more likely to have a recurrence and have to be followed up. Conservative treatment for this group has a lot of disadvantages, and the recommended treatment is surgical- arthroscopic or open—based on current findings. Post-reduction/post-op protocol should include a series of exercises focused on stability of the joint, range of motion and return to play.

Acknowledgements

Parts of this chapter were previously published in the doctoral thesis by the same author: (Svetoslav Dobrilov). Genetic characterisation of (doctor of medicine,

Orthopaedics and Traumatology) (2018). Thesis: "Osteoplastic reconstruction in anterior glenohumeral instability with acquired glenoid bone loss". Medical University "Prof. Dr. Paraskev Stoyanov" Varna, Bulgaria. Available from: (https://www.mu-varna.bg/BG/Research/svetoslav-l-dobrilov-doctor).

Author details

Svetoslav Dobrilov
University Hospital "St. Marina", Varna, Bulgaria

*Address all correspondence to: svetlyo_d@yahoo.com

References

[1] Cooper DE, Arnoczky SP, O'Brien SJ, et al. Anatomy, histology and vascularity of the glenoid labrum: An anatomical study. Journal of Bone and Joint Surgery. 1992;**74-A**:46-52

[2] Boileau P, Walch G. Glenoid slope in osteoarthritic and rheumatoid shoulders before and after arthroplasty. Journal of Shoulder and Elbow Surgery. 1997;**6**:194-195

[3] Roberts SB, Beattie N, McNiven ND, Robinson CM. The natural history of primary anterior dislocation of the glenohumeral joint in adolescence. The Bone & Joint Journal. 2015;**97-B**(4):520-526

[4] Slaa RL, Brand R, Marti RK, et al. A prospective arthroscopic study of acute first-time anterior shoulder dislocation in the young: A five year follow-up study. Journal of Shoulder and Elbow Surgery. 2003;**12**:529-534

[5] Davy AR, Steve JD. Management of shoulder dislocation—Are we doing enough to reduce the risk of recurrence? Injury. 2002;**33**(9):775-779

[6] Robinson CM, Dobson RJ. Anterior instability of the shoulder after trauma. Journal of Bone and Joint Surgery. 2004;**86**(4):469-479

[7] Owens BD, Nelson BJ, Duffey ML, et al. Pathoanatomy of first-time, traumatic, anterior glenohumeral subluxation events. The Journal of Bone and Joint Surgery. American Volume. 2010;**92**:1605-1611

[8] Shields DW, Jefferies JG, Brooksbank AJ, et al. Epidemiology of glenohumeral dislocation and subsequent instability in an urban population. Journal of Shoulder and Elbow Surgery. 2018;**27**:189-195

[9] Brownson P, Donaldson O, Fox M, et al. BESS/BOA patient care pathways: Traumatic anterior shoulder instability. Shoulder and Elbow. 2015;**7**:214-226

[10] Holvelius L, Augustini BG, Fredin H, et al. Primary anterior dislocation of the shoulder in young patients (a ten-year prospective study). Journal of Bone and Joint Surgery. 1996;**78**:1677-1684

[11] Bigliani LU, Newton PM, Steinmann SP, et al. Glenoid rim lesions associated with recurrent anterior dislocation of the shoulder. The American Journal of Sports Medicine. 1998;**26**:41-455

[12] Leroux T, Wasserstein D, Veillette C, et al. Epidemiology of primary anterior shoulder dislocation requiring closed reduction in Ontario, Canada. The American Journal of Sports Medicine. 2014;**42**:442-450

[13] Owens BD, Agel J, Mountcastle SB, et al. Incidence of glenohumeral instability in collegiate athletics. The American Journal of Sports Medicine. 2009;**37**:1750-1754

[14] Sugaya H, Moriishi J, Dohi M. Glenoid rim morphology inrecurrent anterior glenohumeral instability. The Journal of Bone and Joint Surgery. American Volume. 2003;**85**:878-884

[15] Yiannakopoulos CK, Mataragas E, Antonogiannakis E. A comparison of the spectrum of intra-articular lesions in acute and chronic anterior shoulder instability. Arthroscopy. 2007;**23**:985-990

[16] Chapus V, Rochcongar G, Pineau V, et al. Ten-year follow-up of

acute arthroscopic Bankart repair for initial anterior shoulder dislocation in young patients. Orthopaedics & Traumatology, Surgery & Research. 2015;**101**:889-893. DOI: 10.1016/j.otsr.2015.09.029

[17] Baker CL, Uribe JW, Whitman C. Arthroscopic evaluation of acute initial anterior shoulder dislocations. The American Journal of Sports Medicine. 1990;**18**:25-28

[18] Larrain MV, Botto GJ, Montenegro HJ, Mauas DM. Arthroscopic repair of acute traumatic anterior shoulder dislocation in young adults. Arthroscopy. 2001;**17**:373-377

[19] Neviaser TJ. The anterior labroligamentous periosteal sleeve avulsion lesion: A cause of anterior instability of the shoulder. Arthroscopy. 1993;**9**:17-21

[20] Walch G, Boileau P, Levigne C, et al. Arthroscopic stabilisation for recurrent anterior shoulder dislocation: Results of 59 cases. Arthroscopy. 1999;**11**:173-179

[21] Arciero RA, Taylor DC, Snyder RJ, et al. Arthroscopic transglenoid multiple suture repair: 2 to 8 year results in 150 shoulders. Arthroscopy. 1997;**13**:609-619

[22] Neviaser TJ. The GLAD lesion: Another cause of anterior shoulder pain. Arthroscopy. 1993;**9**:22-23

[23] Snyder SJ, Karzel RP, Del Pizzo W, Ferkel RD. Friedman MJ SLAP lesions of the shoulder. Arthroscopy. 1990;**6**:274-279

[24] Warner JJP, Kann S, Marks P. Arthroscopic repair of combined Bankart and superior labral detachment anterior and posterior lesions: Technique and preliminary results. Arthroscopy. 1994;**10**:383-391

[25] Maffet MW, Gartzman GM. Superior labrum-biceps tendon complex lesions of the shoulder. The American Journal of Sports Medicine. 1995;**23**:93-98

[26] Spoor AB, de Waal MJ. Long-term results and arthropathy following the modified Bristow-Latarjet procedure. International Orthopaedics. 2005;**29**(265):7

[27] Wolf EM, Cheng JC, Dickson K. Humeral avulsion of glenohumeral ligaments as a cause of anterior shoulder instability. Arthroscopy. 1995;**11**:600-607

[28] Bui-Mansfield LT, Banks KP, Taylor DC. Humeral avulsion of the glenohumeral ligaments: The HAGL lesion. The American Journal of Sports Medicine. 2007;**35**(11):1960-1966

[29] Itoi E, Tabata S. Rotator cuff tears in anterior dislocation of the shoulder. International Orthopaedics. 1992;**16**:240-244

[30] Burkhart SS, De Beer JF. Traumatic glenohumeral bone defects and their relationship to failure of arthroscopic Bankart repairs: Significance of the inverted-pear glenoid and the humeral engaging Hill–Sachs lesion. Arthroscopy. 2000;**16**:677-694

[31] Chen AL, Hunt SA, Hawkins RJ, Zuckerman JD. Management of bone loss associated with recurrent anterior glenohumeral instability. The American Journal of Sports Medicine. 2005;**33**:912-925

[32] Edwards TB, Boulahia A, Walch G. Radiographic analysis of bone defects in chronic anterior shoulder instability. Arthroscopy. 2003;**19**:732-739

[33] Griffith JF, Antonio GE, Yung PS, et al. Prevalence, pattern, and spectrum of glenoid bone loss in anterior shoulder

dislocation: CT analysis of 218 patients. AJR. American Journal of Roentgenology. 2008;**190**:1247-1254

[34] Griffith J, Antonio G, Tong C, Ming C. Anterior shoulder dislocation: Quantification of glenoid bone loss with CT. American Journal of Roentgenology. 2003;**180**:1423-1430

[35] Franceschi F, Longo UG, Ruzzini L, Rizzello G, Maffulli N, Denaro V. Arthroscopic salvage of failed arthroscopic Bankart repair: A prospective study with a minimum follow-up of 4 years. The American Journal of Sports Medicine. 2008;**36**:1330-1336

[36] Antonio GE, Griffith JF, Yu AB, et al. First-time shoulder dislocation: High prevalence of labral injury and age-related differences revealed by MR arthrography. Journal of Magnetic Resonance Imaging. 2007;**26**:983-991

[37] Bollier MJ, Arciero R. Management of glenoid and humeral bone loss. Sports Medicine and Arthroscopy. 2010;**18**:140-148

[38] Kim DS, Yoon YS, Yi CH. Prevalence comparison of accompanying lesions between primary and recurrent anterior dislocation in the shoulder. The American Journal of Sports Medicine. 2010;**38**:2071-2076

[39] Greis PE, Scuderi MG, Mohr A, Bachus KN, Burks RT. Glenohumeral articular contact areas and pressures following labral and osseous injury to the anteroinferior quadrant of the glenoid. Journal of Shoulder and Elbow Surgery. 2002;**11**:442-451

[40] Mologne TS, Provencher MT, Menzel KA, et al. Arthroscopic stabilisation in patients with an inverted pear glenoid: Results in patients with bone loss of the anterior glenoid. The American Journal of Sports Medicine. 2007;**35**:1276-1283

[41] Boileau P, Villalba M, Hery JY, Balg F, Ahrens P, et al. Risk factors for recurrence of shoulder instability after arthroscopic Bankart repair. The Journal of Bone and Joint Surgery. American Volume. 2006;**88**:1755-1763

[42] Sugaya H, Moriishi J, Kanisawa I, Tsuchiya A. Arthroscopic osseous Bankart repair for chronic recurrent traumatic anterior glenohumeral instability. The Journal of Bone and Joint Surgery. American Volume. 2005;**87**:1752-1760

[43] Kardouni JR, McKinnon CJ, Seitz AL. Incidence of shoulder dislocations and the rate of recurrent instability in soldiers. Medicine and Science in Sports and Exercise. 2016;**48**:2150-2156

[44] Vermeiren J, Handelberg F, Casteleyn PP, Opdecam P. The rate of recurrence of traumatic anterior dislocation of the shoulder. A study of 154 cases and a review of the literature. International Orthopaedics. 1993;**17**:337-341

[45] Bigliani LU, Newton PM, Steinmann SP, et al. Glenoid rim lesions associated with recurrent anterior dislocation of the shoulder Am. The Journal of Sports Medicine. 1998;**26**:41-455

[46] Ji JH, Kwak DS, Yang PS, et al. Comparisons of glenoid bony defects between normal cadaveric specimens and patients with recurrent shoulder dislocation: An anatomic study. Journal of Shoulder and Elbow Surgery. 2012;**21**(6):822-827

[47] Saito H, Itoi E, Sugaya H, et al. Location of the glenoid defect in shoulders with recurrent anterior

dislocation. The American Journal of Sports Medicine. 2005;**33**:889-893

[48] Yamamoto N, Itoi E, Abe H, et al. Contact between the glenoid and the humeral head in abduction, external rotation, and horizontal extension: A new concept of glenoid track. Journal of Shoulder and Elbow Surgery. 2007;**16**:649-656.15

[49] Kaar S, Fening S, Jones M, Colbrunn R, Miniaci A. Effect of humeral head defect size on glenohumeral stability: A cadaveric study of simulated Hill-Sachs defects. The American Journal of Sports Medicine. 2010;**38**(3):594-599

[50] Sekiya JK, Jolly J, Debski RE. The effect of a Hill-Sachs defect on glenohumeral translations, in situ capsular forces, and bony contact forces. The American Journal of Sports Medicine. 2012;**40**(2):388-394

[51] Randelli P, Ragone V, Carminati S, Cabitza P. Risk factorsfor recurrence after Bankart repair a systematic review. Knee Surgery, Sports Traumatology, Arthroscopy. 2012;**20**:2129-2138

[52] Imhoff AB, Ansah P, Tischer T, Reiter C, Bartl C, et al. Arthroscopic repair of anterior-inferior glenohumeral instability using a portal at the 5:30-o'clock position: Analysis of the effects of age, fixation method, and concomitant shoulder injury on surgical outcomes. The American Journal of Sports Medicine. 2010;**38**(9):1795-1803

[53] Jobe FW, Kvitne RS, Giangarra CE. Shoulder pain in the overhand or throwing athlete: The relationship of anterior instability and rotator cuff impingement. Orthopaedic Review. 1989;**18**:963-975

[54] Farber AJ, Castillo R, Bahk M, McFarland E. Clinical assessment of three commont tests for traumatic anteriror shoulder instability. The Journal of Bone and Joint Surgery. 2006;**88**:1467-1474

[55] Chuang TY, Adam CR, Burkhart SS. Use of preoperative three-dimensional computed tomography to quantify glenoid bone loss in shoulder instability. Arthroscopy. 2008;**24**:376-382

[56] Hayes ML, Collins MS, Morgan JA, Wenger DE, Dahm DL. Efficacy of diagnostic magnetic resonanceimaging for articular cartilage lesions of the glenohumeral joint in patients with instability. Skeletal Radiology. 2010;**39**:1199-1204

[57] Zanetti M, Weishaupt D, Jost B, Gerber C, Hodler J. MR imaging for traumatic tears of the rotator cuff: High prevalence of greater tuberosity fractures and subscapularis tendon tears. AJR. 1999;**172**:463-446

[58] Alkaduhimi H, van der Linde JA, Flipsen M, van Deurzen DFP, van den Bekerom MPJ. A systematic and technical guide on how to reduce a shoulder dislocation. Turkish Journal of Emergency Medicine. 2016;**16**:155-168

[59] Hatamabadi HR, Arhami Dolatabadi A, Derakhshanfar H, Younesian S, Ghaffari Shad E. Propofol versus midazolam for procedural sedation of anterior shoulder dislocation in emergency department: A randomized clinical trial. Trauma Monthly. 2015;**20**(2):e13530

[60] Smith BI, Bliven KCH, Morway GR, Hurbanek JG. Management of primary anterior shoulder dislocations using immobilization. Journal of Athletic Training. 2015;**50**:550-552

[61] Itoi E, Sashi R, Minagawa H, Shimizu T, Wakabayashi I, Sato K. Position of immobilization after

dislocation of the glenohumeral joint. A study with use of magnetic resonance imaging. The Journal of Bone and Joint Surgery. American Volume. 2001;**83-A**:661-667

[62] Maeda A, Yoneda M, Horibe S, Hirooka A, Wakitani S, Narita Y. Longer immobilization extends the "symptom-free" period following primary shoulder dislocation in young rugby players. Journal of Orthopaedic Science. 2002;**7**(1):43-47

[63] Paterson WH, Throckmorton TW, Koester M, Azar FM, Kuhn JE. Position and duration of immobilization after primary anterior shoulder dislocation: A systematic review and meta-analysis of the literature. The Journal of Bone and Joint Surgery. American Volume. 2010;**92**(18):2924-2933

[64] Robinson CM, Howes J, Murdoch H, Will E, Graham C. Functional outcome and risk of recurrent instability after primary traumatic anterior shoulder dislocation in young patients. The Journal of Bone and Joint Surgery. American Volume. 2006;**88**(11):2326-2336

[65] Murray IR, Ahmed I, White NJ, Robinson CM. Traumatic anterior shoulder instability in the athlete. Scandinavian Journal of Medicine & Science in Sports. 2013;**23**(4):387-405

[66] Hurley ET, Jamal MS, Ali ZS, Montgomery C, Pauzenberger L, Mullett H. Long-term outcomes of the Latarjet procedure for anterior shoulder instability: A systematic review of studies at 10-year follow-up. Journal of Shoulder and Elbow Surgery. 2019;**28**:e33-e39

[67] Aboalata M, Plath JE, Seppel G, Juretzko J, Vogt S, et al. Results of arthroscopic Bankart repair for anterior-inferior shoulder instability at 13-year follow-up. The American Journal of Sports Medicine. 2017;**45**:782-787

Chapter 4

Scapular Glenoid Fractures

Shuming Huang, Shuhua Lan, Panpan Xie and Jiekai Ye

Abstract

This chapter provides a comprehensive overview of glenoid fractures, including their epidemiology, injury mechanism, anatomy and biomechanics, clinical examination, imaging methods, classifications of fractures, diagnosis and treatment options, rehabilitation, and complications. The management of scapular glenoid fractures should be individualized according to fracture characteristics (type/clock orientation), patient factors, and the surgeon's expertise. While most scapular fractures achieve favorable outcomes with conservative management, surgical intervention is recommended for glenoid-involved fractures, particularly those with significant displacement that may lead to post-traumatic arthritis or glenohumeral instability. Introduction of various surgical approaches with clinical cases, such as classical approaches, modified approaches (mini-open anterior approach, posterior "safe zone" approach), and merging approaches (axillary approach, arthroscopy-assisted technique, etc.). This chapter emphasizes the importance of patient-centered care and highlights evolving strategies to optimize treatment outcomes.

Keywords: scapula fracture, scapular glenoid, surgical approach, axillary approach, shoulder joint, fracture fixation, internal, glenoid fixation

1. Introduction

Shoulder joint stability is crucial for both daily function and athletic performance. As a critical component of this joint, the structural integrity of the scapular glenoid significantly influences overall shoulder function and stability [1]. Glenoid fractures, particularly those associated with shoulder instability, have become a focal point in clinical research. However, the mechanisms of injury, fracture morphology, and optimal treatment strategies for these fractures are still not fully understood. While most scapular fractures achieve favorable outcomes with conservative management, displaced glenoid fractures require surgical fixation to avoid complications such as malunion, post-traumatic glenohumeral osteoarthritis, chronic instability, and persistent pain [2, 3]. Thus, accurate diagnosis, comprehensive assessment, and appropriate management are critical in addressing these injuries.

2. Epidemiology and etiology

Scapular fractures represent a relatively rare injury, with current epidemiological data on glenoid fractures remaining sparse. Reported incidence rates vary considerably across different populations and clinical settings. Scapular fractures constitute approximately 1.7% of all fractures in the adult population, according to the US National Trauma Data Bank data [4]. The occurrence of glenoid rim and intra-articular glenoid fractures ranges from 28.4 to 48.5% of all scapular fractures [5, 6]. The increasing diagnosis of glenoid fractures over the past decade mirrors both population aging trends and the utilization of CT imaging in clinical practice [4]. Most glenoid fractures occur secondary to high-energy trauma, with young and middle-aged adults being predominantly affected. A significant male predominance is observed, likely reflecting greater male engagement in high-risk activities and consequent increased exposure to high-energy trauma mechanisms [6]. And low-energy fall injuries have become the main mechanism of injury in the elderly population.

The injury mechanisms underlying scapular glenoid fossa fractures remain incompletely characterized. However, current evidence suggests that the majority of glenoid fossa fractures result from direct impaction of the humeral head against the articular surface. Avulsion fractures and glenoid rim fractures are strongly associated with shoulder dislocations and subsequent instability, with sports injuries and falls being the predominant etiological factors [7]. Complex scapular glenoid fractures typically result from high-energy trauma such as motor vehicle traffic accidents, bicycle accidents, and falls from height. The injury mechanism involves either direct impact or indirect force transmission through the humeral head, with fracture patterns determined by the glenoid contact point and force vector at impact [1].

In scaphoid fractures, neighboring skeletal structures are susceptible to fracture as a result of similar high-energy traumatic external forces. Multiple large database studies have reported that 21–50% of scaphoid fractures occur in conjunction with at least one concomitant injury [5, 6, 8]. Common concomitant injuries include rib fractures, pulmonary contusions, hemopneumothorax, pneumonia, clavicle fractures, proximal humerus fractures, traumatic brain injuries, and spinal fractures [4, 5]. Among glenoid fractures, associated clavicle fractures occur in 2.8% of cases, while proximal humerus fractures are seen in 8.3% of cases (**Figure 1**) [6].

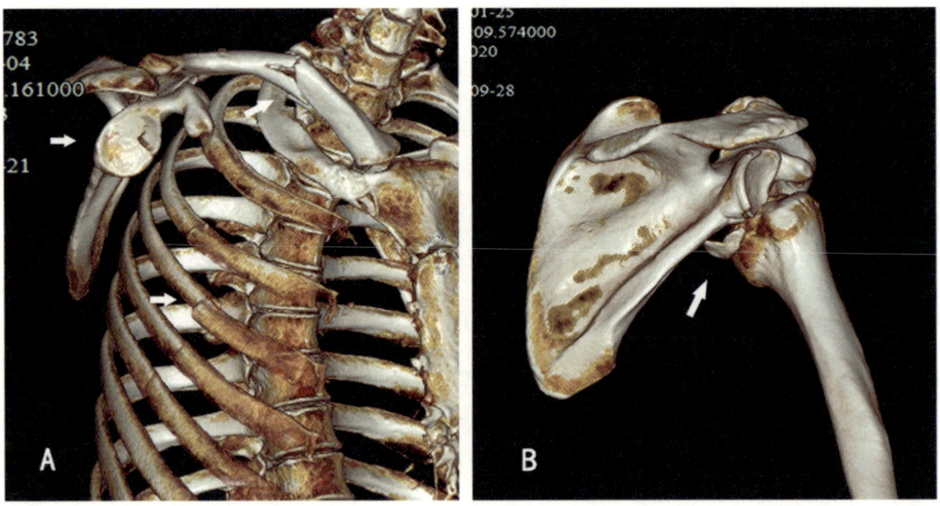

Figure 1.
Glenoid fractures with associated injuries. (A) Glenoid fracture accompanied by clavicular fracture and multiple rib fractures. (B) Glenoid fracture with anterior shoulder dislocation and humeral head fracture (Hill-Sachs lesion).

3. Anatomy and biomechanics

The glenoid fossa (or cavity), a shallow articular depression on the lateral aspect of the scapula, forms a synovial ball-and-socket joint with the humeral head [9]. The fossa's depth is reinforced by a variable-thickness, ring-shaped fibrocartilaginous glenoid labrum that circumferentially surrounds the osseous rim [10]. The average surface area of the articular glenoid cartilage is 5.6 cm^2 in males and 4.7 cm^2 in females, and the average thickness of the articular cartilage of the scapular glenoid is 3.8 mm [11]. The cartilage partially compensates for the instability of the shoulder joint, and the fibrous labrum surrounding the glenoid cavity further enhances the congruence of the joint.

The scapular glenoid fossa can be systematically described and localized using two principal anatomical reference methods. The first employs a clock-face orientation, where the 12 o'clock position corresponds to the superior aspect and 3 o'clock to the anterior aspect. The alternative approach divides the fossa into four anatomical quadrants: superior, anterior, inferior, and posterior regions [10]. When viewed in the face, the glenoid articular surface demonstrates a characteristic biphasic morphology consisting of two overlapping circular structures: a smaller superior portion and a larger inferior surface (**Figure 2**). Studies have shown that the shape of the glenoid cavity varies among individuals and can be categorized into three main types: pear-shaped, inverted comma-shaped, and oval [12, 13]. These shape differences are closely related to the notch on the anterosuperior edge of the glenoid cavity. The mean glenoid anteroposterior diameter is 24.7 ± 3.5 mm, and the mean glenoid height is 31.7 ± 3.7 mm, with the glenoid height and width being larger in males than in females [14].

The glenoid fossa's relatively flat and diminutive articular surface, articulating with 33% of the humeral head in any position, enables the shoulder's remarkable range of motion at the expense of inherent stability [7, 9]. Therefore, the

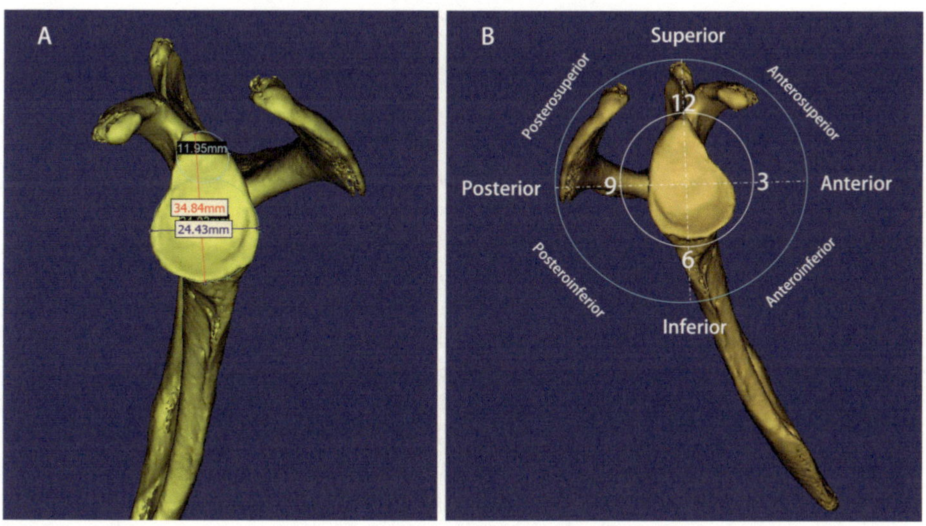

Figure 2.
Anatomical morphology and anatomical location description of the scapular glenoid fossa. (A) Biphasic glenoid morphology demonstrating overlapping circular structures, with annotated measurements of anteroposterior diameter and glenoid height. (B) The clock-face orientation and four anatomical quadrants approach are used to illustrate the location of glenoid fossa fractures.

glenohumeral joint requires coordinated action between its static and dynamic stabilizers to preserve proper congruity and functionality. The static stabilizers of the glenohumeral joint comprise the articular anatomy (glenoid and humeral head), fibrocartilaginous labrum, the articular capsule, negative intra-articular pressure, and the superior, middle, and inferior glenohumeral ligaments. Static stabilizers play a crucial role, as their isolated injury can lead to recurrent instability. The primary dynamic stabilizers of the glenohumeral joint are the musculotendinous components, including the rotator cuff muscles: supraspinatus, infraspinatus, subscapularis, and teres minor. These muscles function as a force couple, maintaining humeral head centration within the glenoid fossa during movement [10, 15].

4. Clinical assessment and imaging methods

Glenoid fracture patients characteristically manifest localized pain, restricted shoulder movement, and aggravated pain with abduction. Nearly half of scaphoid fracture patients present with concomitant injuries, frequently including pulmonary contusion, pneumothorax/hemothorax, craniocerebral trauma, and other fractures [5]. Similarly, glenoid fossa fractures are frequently associated with concomitant injuries, including thoracic trauma, head injuries, brachial plexus involvement, shoulder dislocation, and multiple humeral fractures. Thus, surgeons should remain vigilant for potential accompanying injuries and ensure that all patients undergo a systematic clinical evaluation to minimize missed diagnoses and enable prompt resuscitation. A comprehensive examination of the shoulder girdle must include inspection for soft tissue injuries, such as abrasions, open wounds, and degloving injuries [16]. These findings can significantly influence surgical decision-making regarding timing and risk assessment. Meanwhile, a focused shoulder examination should encompass the active and passive range of motion, strength testing, and neurovascular assessment [1]. Most patients are unable to perform a motor strength assessment of the shoulder because of pain and can only examine and record whether the innervation area is normal.

Imaging is critical for diagnosing and classifying glenoid fractures, directly guiding clinical management. If a scapular glenoid fracture is suspected, initial evaluation should consider including an appropriate set of radiograph series (**Figure 3**): (1) anterior-posterior (AP), (2) anteroposterior oblique (Grashey view) or sometimes referred to as true AP, (3) lateral (scapula Y view), (4) axillary view, and (5) apical oblique view [17–19]. The true anteroposterior (Grashey) view, apical oblique view, and axillary view are particularly valuable for visualizing intra-articular fractures of the glenoid fossa and rim, as well as dislocations within the glenohumeral joint cavity. Similarly, it is indispensable to assess the quality of fracture reduction and ensure that the internal fixation hardware is positioned outside the articular surface.

In clinical practice, Computed Tomography (CT) plays a critical role in assessing glenoid fractures by providing detailed visualization of fracture characteristics. This enables precise evaluation and clear visualization of fracture morphology, including the fragment size, location, degree of displacement, and position of the humeral glenoid joint [20]. Consequently, it aids orthopedic surgeons in accurate fracture classification and informs optimal treatment strategies. For complex scapular fractures involving the glenoid fossa, digital subtraction of the humeral head from three-dimensional reconstructed imaging data often enables a more intuitive assessment of

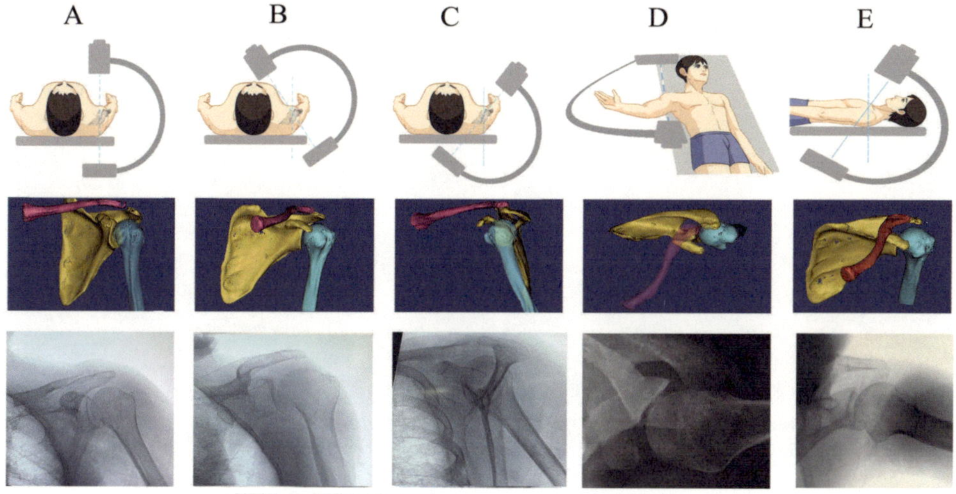

Figure 3.
X-ray plain film series. (A) Anterior-posterior (AP) view of the shoulder. The beam of projection is perpendicular to the torso but oblique to the glenohumeral joint. (B) AP oblique (Grashey view), as a true AP view of the scapula. The projection beam is angled 35–45 degrees toward the healthy side to achieve overlapping of the anterior and posterior glenoid margins, forming a single arcuate line. (C) Lateral (scapula Y view). (D) Axillary view (superior-inferior axial view of the glenohumeral joint) visualizes anterior/posterior glenoid rims while helping in the assessment of glenohumeral instability and dislocation. (E) The apical oblique view, which is a modification of the axillary projection, offers a unique perspective for visualizing the anterior and inferior aspects of the glenoid rim. The X-ray beam traverses the glenohumeral joint with a dual 45° angulation, medially relative to the thoracic plane and caudally toward the detector.

the articular surface, providing complete visualization of the glenoid cavity. While CT remains primary for fracture characterization, Magnetic Resonance Imaging (MRI) should be considered when evaluating for: (1) articular cartilage injury or labral lesion, (2) rotator cuff tear, or (3) ligamentous instability associated with glenoid fractures (**Figure 4**) [21].

5. Classification

The Goss-modified Ideberg classification, which describes six fracture types, is the most widely used system in the literature [22, 23]. Type I is a glenoid rim fracture, subdivided into:Ia (anterior rim, "Bony Bankart"), the most common glenoid fracture, typically associated with shoulder dislocation; Ib (posterior rim). Type II involves an inferior glenoid fracture extending into the neck region, frequently resulting in humeral head subluxation. Type III consists of a transverse superior glenoid fossa fracture extending superomedially through the coracoid base, typically involving the superior shoulder suspensory complex. Type IV fractures extend horizontally through the glenoid cavity into the scapular body. Type V is based on type IV injuries with different combinations of the previous fractures and is divided into three combination subtypes of fractures Va (II + IV), Vb (III + IV), and Vc (II + III + IV). Type VI is a comminuted fracture of the articular glenoid (**Figure 5**).

The Arbeitsgemeinschaft für Osteosynthesefragen Foundation and the Orthopedic Trauma Association (AO/OTA) categorize glenoid fractures into two main types: 14F1

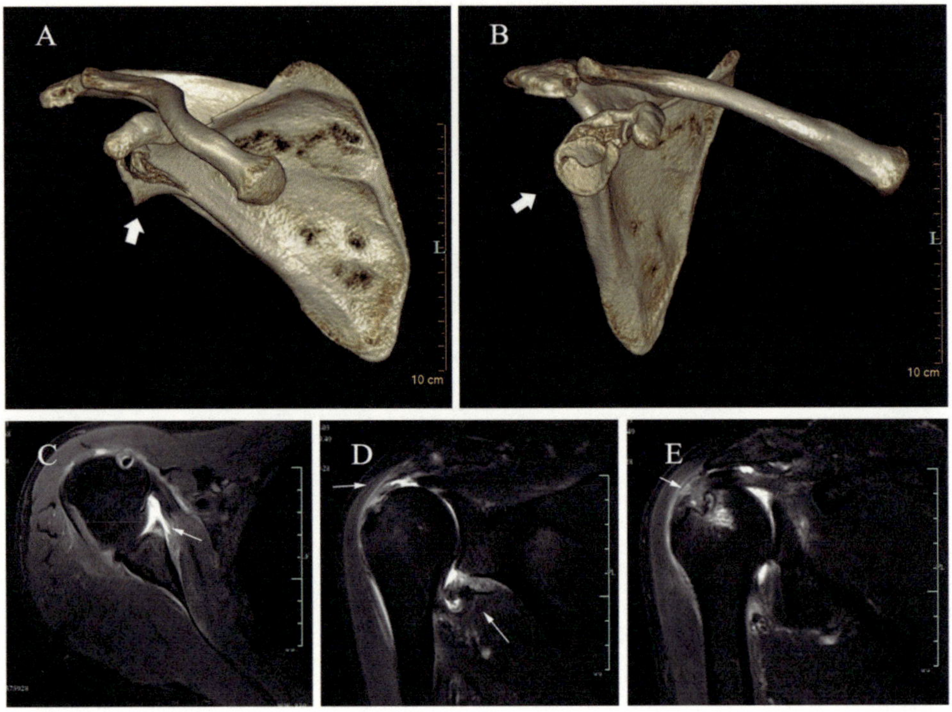

Figure 4.
3D CT with digital subtraction of the humeral head and MRI for comprehensive shoulder injury assessment. (A, B) 3D CT reconstruction with humeral head subtraction visualizing a comminuted glenoid fracture from different perspectives. (C) A case of postreduction Hill-Sachs lesion following closed reduction of shoulder dislocation. Axial T2-weighted MRI demonstrates an anterior-inferior glenoid labral fracture, and capsule elongation with associated fluid signal. (D, E) Coronal T2-weighted MRI shows an anterior-inferior glenoid labral fracture, rotator cuff tear, and depressed fracture of the apex of the humeral head.

(simple intra-articular fractures with a single fracture line) and 14F2 (comminuted intra-articular fractures) [24]. The 14F1 type includes anterior rim fractures (14F1.1) with three subtypes (f: isolated infraequatorial; r: biequatorial crossing the glenoid equator; t: combined anterior-posterior infraequatorial), posterior rim fractures (14F1.2) with three subtypes, and transverse/short oblique fractures (14F1.3) classified by horizontal position (i: infraequatorial; e: equatorial; p: supraequatorial). The 14F2 type is subdivided based on the presence of three or more articular fragments with or without central fracture-dislocation (**Figure 6**).

Bartoníček currently proposes five fundamental types of scapular glenoid fractures, which are identified through the analysis of three-dimensional CT scans: superior, anterior, posterior, inferior, and complete glenoid fractures. Among them, the inferior glenoid fracture is the most prevalent, comprising 42% of all articular glenoid fossa fractures [25]. The Ideberg-Goss classification, featuring a six-type categorization of glenoid rim and fossa fractures, continues to be the preferred system in clinical practice. However, Gilbert has recently shown that the AO/OTA classification system offers greater clinical utility than the Ideberg system. In their study evaluating 84 scapular glenoid fractures, they found that 25% (21/84) could not be classified using the Ideberg criteria. In contrast, the AO/OTA system is more suitable for a valid, reliable, and consistent description of scapular glenoid fractures [26].

DOI: http://dx.doi.org/10.5772/intechopen.1011353

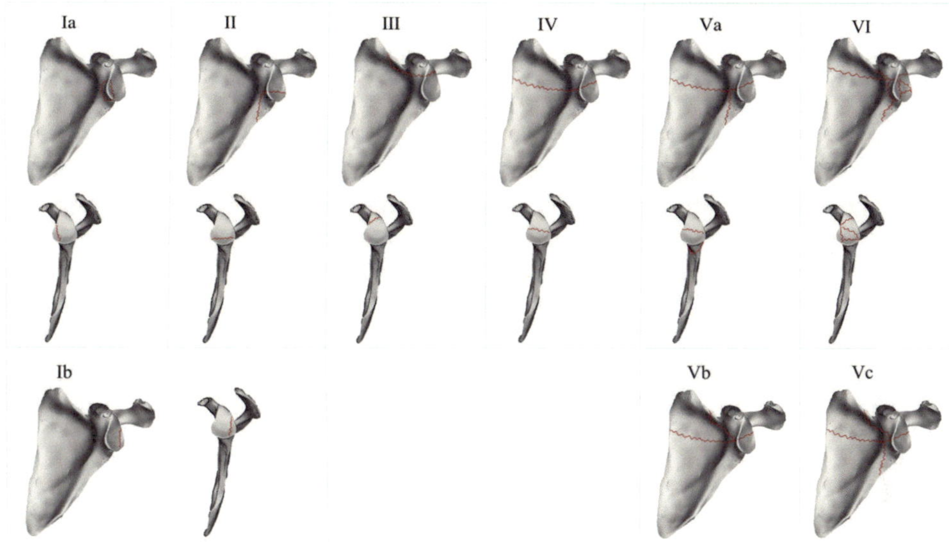

Figure 5.
Illustrative representation of the Ideberg-Goss classification system for glenoid fractures [22, 23].

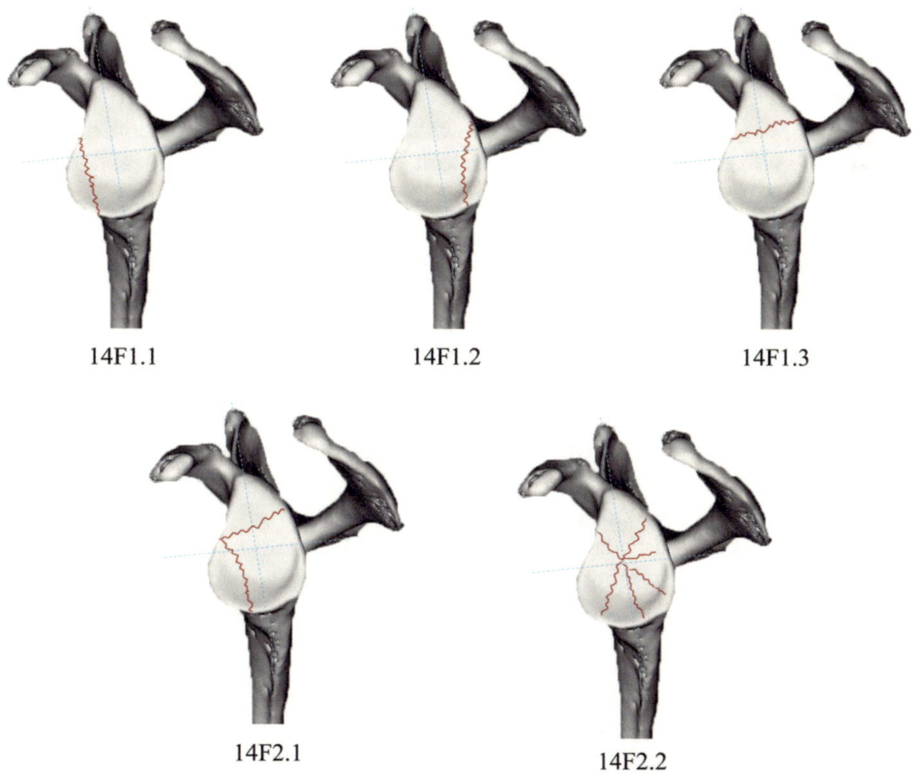

Figure 6.
AO/OTA classification of glenoid fractures [24]. F1, simple glenoid fossa fractures; F2, multi-fragmentary glenoid fossa fractures.

6. Treatment

6.1 Nonoperative management and indications

The majority of scapular body and neck fractures can be treated conservatively, in addition to sufficient displacement and angulation, generally achieving bony union with good functional outcomes and eventual return to work [27, 28]. In contrast, nonoperative management of intra-articular glenoid fractures yields the poorest functional outcomes, with patients frequently experiencing persistent pain, limited shoulder mobility, and diminished strength. The most common complications are poor fracture healing, recurrent shoulder instability necessitating surgical intervention, and post-traumatic osteoarthritis [27, 29]. As a result, glenoid rim and glenoid fossa fractures are more likely to require surgical intervention. However, those glenoid fractures that are very small or minimally displaced with stability and congruity of the glenohumeral joint can be treated conservatively [29, 30]. Initial management involves 4–6 weeks of sling immobilization followed by supervised physiotherapy [9, 31]. Due to the inherent risk of displacement and malunion, weekly or biweekly radiographic monitoring is essential during this critical period.

In the management of glenoid fractures, treatment decisions are guided by fragment size, the degree of displacement, chronicity, and patient activity level, as these factors critically influence the stability, congruity, and concentricity of the glenohumeral joint. The relationship between glenoid bone loss and glenohumeral instability has long been recognized and is widely accepted in the field of orthopedics. Instability is likely to occur with displaced anterior rim fractures that exceed 20–25% of the articular surface, or when the posterior articular surface involvement is more than 33% [32]. Recent research shows that 52% of first-time shoulder instability incidents involve over 5% glenoid bone loss, and nearly 20% of initial dislocations feature rim fractures, resulting in bone loss exceeding 13.5% [33].

Patients with low activity levels and small displaced glenoid rim fractures of less than 5% are usually considered to be treated nonoperatively [1, 34]. However, some studies suggest that consideration of glenohumeral instability as a problem should not be based exclusively on the size of the fragments, but rather on the alignment of the joint after glenoid fracture [31, 35]. The current evidence base lacks comprehensive comparative studies establishing definitive criteria for surgical versus conservative management of glenoid fractures, creating uncertainty in clinical decision-making pathways (**Figure** 7). In many studies, a displacement (fracture gap) or intra-articular step-off of glenoid fractures exceeding 4 mm or 5 mm has been used as an indication for surgery [29, 30, 32, 36]. Additionally, surgical intervention should also be considered in cases of glenoid fracture accompanied by humeral head displacement or subluxation, particularly when two or more injuries to the superior shoulder suspensory complex (SSSC) are present.

6.2 Surgical approaches

The primary goals of glenoid fracture surgery are to restore articular congruity, enhance joint stability, minimize post-traumatic osteoarthritis, and facilitate early functional recovery—thereby preventing shoulder stiffness and improving mobility. Surgical management typically involves either open reduction and internal fixation (ORIF) or arthroscopic-assisted reduction followed by stabilization using suture anchors and screws.

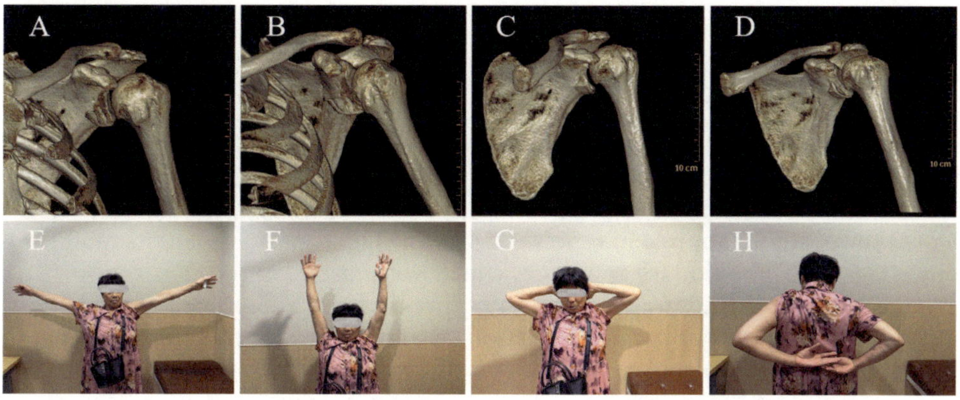

Figure 7.
A 71-year-old female patient with a left anterior-inferior glenoid fracture of the injury who recovered satisfactorily after nonoperative treatment. (A, B) Photographs of 3D CT reconstruction demonstrate a large, displaced glenoid rim fragment after injury. (C, D) CT scans reveal stability, congruity, and concentricity of the glenohumeral joint, partial reduction, and union at 6 months after the injury. (E–H) Photographs show the patient with free active overhead function, active external rotation, and active internal rotation, pain-free.

6.2.1 Arthroscopic techniques

Modern advancements in arthroscopic techniques and instrumentation have made it possible to treat many glenoid fractures with minimally invasive repair procedures. Arthroscopy provides the advantages of minimized soft tissue dissection, reduced surgical trauma, and more accurate fracture reduction of the glenoid through direct visualization. Additionally, this technique enables simultaneous diagnosis and treatment of concomitant shoulder injuries, including rotator cuff tears and glenoid labral injuries (**Figure 8**). However, this technique requires the orthopedic surgeon to have substantial experience in shoulder arthroscopy and entails a steep learning curve. Current literature establishes arthroscopy as a safe and effective treatment option, with predominant application in type I glenoid rim fractures [3, 37–40]. Arthroscopic management has also been successfully reported for Ideberg type II–V glenoid fractures [41–43]. Arthroscopic glenoid fracture management offers three principal fixation options: (1) suture anchor fixation (single- or double-row), (2) transglenoid suture fixation through osseous tunnels (such as Endobutton), and (3) percutaneous screw fixation for larger fragments requiring rigid stabilization [38, 39, 41, 43–45]. The approach is selected based on fracture characteristics, with suture techniques preferred for smaller fragments (<25% articular surface) and screw fixation reserved for larger fragments.

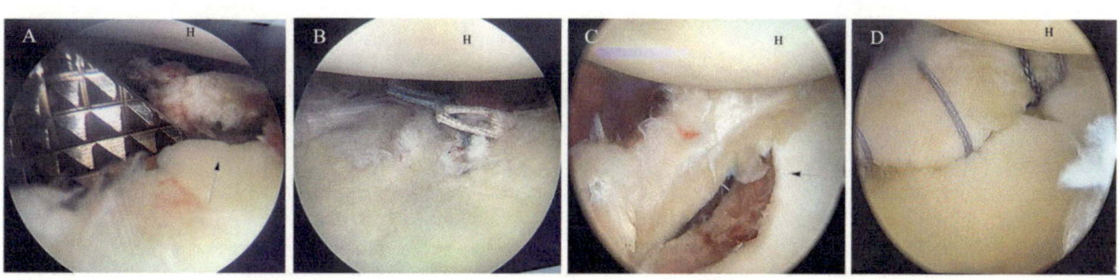

Figure 8.
Arthroscopic views of the glenoid rim fractures (A, C) and the fixed fragment with suture anchors (B, D).

6.2.2 ORIF techniques

Typically, all glenoid fractures are treatable by open approaches. Depending on the type and location of the fracture, various surgical approaches can be employed to visualize and address a displaced glenoid fracture. The more common surgical approaches for glenoid fractures in clinical practice include: (1) the anterior approach, represented by the delto-pectoral approach and its modifications [46, 47]; (2) the posterior approach, represented by the Judet approach and its modifications [48–50]; (3) the axillary approach, which has emerged in recent years [46, 51]. For complex glenoid fractures, surgeons may prefer to use a combined approach or a superior osteotomy approach. Moreover, acromial osteotomy, either alone or in combination with distal clavicular osteotomy, has been documented as effective access strategies for the superior and superior-posterior glenoid (at 10–1 o'clock) and Ideberg VI glenoid fossa fractures in the literature [52, 53]. Definitive fixation following open reduction of glenoid fractures may utilize a variety of options, including various sizes and types of cannulated screws, headless compression screws, plate osteosynthesis, and suture anchor augmentation.

The anterior approach provides optimal exposure for the anterior glenoid in range from the 11- to 6-o'clock orientation. This includes anterior rim fracture (Ideberg Ia), inferior or anterior-inferior fracture (Ideberg II), transverse intra-articular glenoid fossa fracture (Ideberg IV), and superior glenoid fracture involving disruption of the SSSC (Ideberg III) [47, 54]. The patient is positioned supine or in the beach chair position, and the classic delto-pectoral approach is utilized. To achieve an extensive visualization of the anterior glenoid surgical field, the subscapularis muscle is longitudinally split at the myotendinous junction, maintaining a distance of at least 1 cm from the insertion site. After the fracture has been internally fixed, the split subscapularis is sutured with the arm in neutral rotation. However, this approach may limit early external rotation rehabilitation. In addressing Ideberg type III superior glenoid fractures, a supra-subscapularis approach is typically preferred, which avoids muscle splitting while providing adequate exposure for fracture reduction and fixation (**Figure 9**).

The axillary approach for treating Ideberg Ia and II scapular glenoid fractures, particularly inferior and anterior-inferior glenoid rim fractures, offers the advantage of transfracture line and buttress fixation, which can be challenging to achieve with

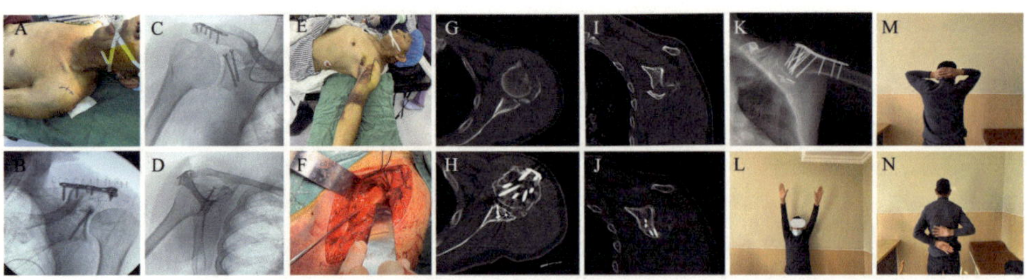

Figure 9.
The glenoid fracture was treated with open reduction and internal fixation via an anterior approach. (A, B) A supra-subscapularis approach was used for an Ideberg type IV glenoid fracture, featuring a small anterior incision while preserving the subscapularis muscle. (C, D) A supra-subscapularis approach was used for an Ideberg type III glenoid fracture. (E, F) The classic delto-pectoral approach was utilized, and the subscapularis muscle was longitudinally split at the myotendinous junction. (G–J) Preoperative and postoperative CT scan images demonstrated an anterior-inferior glenoid fracture combined with a proximal humeral fracture. (K) Postoperative X-ray film. (L–N) Two years after the operation, the patient achieved satisfactory function.

the anterior approach [46, 51, 55]. The patient is positioned in lateral decubitus with the affected shoulder abducted 90°. A 6–8 cm incision begins at the anterior-superior aspect of the axillary fold along the posterior axillary border, extending inferiorly following the anterior margin of the latissimus dorsi. Dissection proceeds bluntly along the anterior border and tendon of the latissimus dorsi, deeply exposing the joint capsule, the axillary border of the scapular neck, and the fracture fragments in the space between the subscapularis and latissimus dorsi tendons. Intraoperatively, it is important to gently move the shoulder joint and use finger touch to find the position of the glenohumeral joint. Also, the axillary nerve and main blood vessels should be carefully identified, separated, and protected (**Figure 10**).

The posterior approach. The original and classic Judet approach provides extensive exposure to the scapular body and the posterior part of the glenoid. This approach is primarily indicated for the surgical treatment of Ideberg type IV and V fractures [48, 56]. Its advantages include adequate visualization of comminuted scapular fractures, the posterior scapular glenoid, and scapular body fractures extending into the scapular glenoid fracture. Additionally, it allows for intraoperative assessment of suprascapular nerve impingement due to suprascapular notch fractures. The patient is positioned laterally or prone. The incision, shaped like a boomerang, begins at the posterior lateral border of the acromion, travels inward along the scapular spine, and then follows the contour of the shoulder. It extends downward along the medial border of the scapula. To visualize the scapular body and the posterior aspect of the glenoid, the posterior deltoid fascicle attached to the scapular spine is divided and separated, and the flap of the infraspinatus muscle is retracted laterally by stripping it from the medial border of the scapula and the subscapular fossa. During the procedure, the suprascapular nerve and artery can be identified and protected in the portion of the posterior superior glenoid corner. While the traditional Judet approach offers extensive exposure, it requires extensive soft tissue dissection, including detachment of both the deltoid and infraspinatus muscles. The modified Judet approach, as described by Obremskey et al., utilizes a similar skin incision to the Judet approach [50]. This approach preserves the infraspinatus muscle by avoiding its detachment, instead accessing the posterior glenoid through the natural plane between the infraspinatus and teres minor muscles, facilitated by a reverse

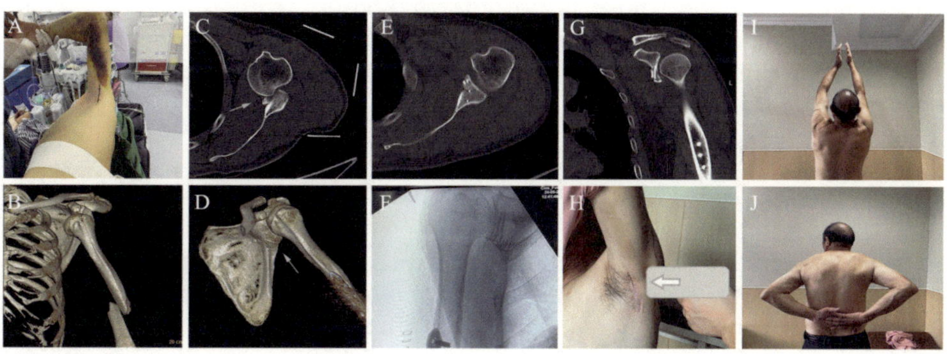

Figure 10.
Glenoid fracture ORIF via *axillary approach. (A) Surgical positioning and incision marking. (B, C) CT images demonstrate a Hill-Sachs injury, an anterior-inferior glenoid fracture, and a humeral shaft fracture. (D) Postoperative 3D-CT following ORIF of humeral fracture and shoulder dislocation reduction. (E–G) Postoperative CT and X-ray images. (H) Surgical scar on the axillary skin. (I, J) Activities of the shoulder joint 6 months after the operation.*

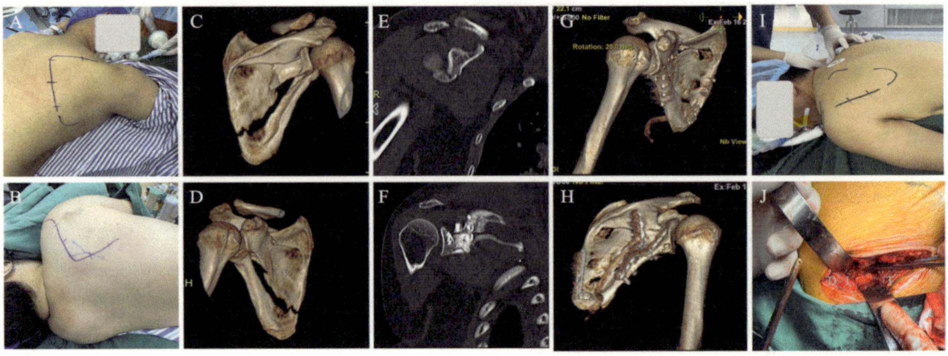

Figure 11.
The posterior approach of the Judet approach and its modification. (A, B) Body markings for Judet approach incisions in prone and supine positions. (C–E) CT images demonstrate Ideberg type IV glenoid fractures and comminuted fractures of the body and spine of the scapula. (F–H) Postoperative 3D-CT following ORIF by Judet approach. (I, J) Postoperative CT and X-ray images. (H) Surgical scar on the axillary skin. (I, J) A small straight incision along the lateral scapular border with posterior deltoid-sparing approach with modified Judet approach.

subcutaneous flap and deltoid retraction. If the goal is solely to treat and visualize the posterior scapular glenoid, a simple modified Judet approach can be considered. A transverse incision is made below the scapular spine. The posterior deltoid fascicle is then dissected off of the spine of the scapula and reflected laterally. Similar to other modified approaches, the posterior glenoid is exposed through the interval between the infraspinatus and teres minor muscles. For complex intra-articular fractures, it may sometimes be necessary to split the infraspinatus muscle near the humeral head and then expand the glenoid fracture by retracting the subscapularis muscle medially to fully expose the glenoid fracture. In addition, for the surgical management of Ideberg type Ib or II fractures, an alternative option is a small straight incision along the lateral scapular border with a posterior deltoid-sparing approach [49]. An 8- to 10-cm straight incision is made along the lateral edge of the scapula. The deltoid fascia is incised and retracted cephalad. Dissection is performed between the infraspinatus and teres minor muscles. The infraspinatus is retracted proximally and the teres minor distally to expose the posterior and posterior-inferior aspects of the glenoid. If the glenoid fracture extends to the medial aspect of the scapular body, internal fixation can be assisted by making a small incision along the medial edge of the glenoid body (**Figure 11**).

7. Rehabilitation and complications

In the postoperative period, rehabilitation management must be tailored to the surgical approach (e.g., open vs. arthroscopic) and intraoperative stability (e.g., the proper bony fragment fixaticty). Generally, the affected shoulder is immobilized in a comfortable sling or abduction pillow sling for 3–4 weeks after surgery with no lifting or bearing weight. Patients initiate passive shoulder exercises under a physical therapist's supervision immediately, within pain tolerance, and continue for 1 month based on fracture fixation stability. Exceptions occurred only when repairing complex rotator cuff tears, specifically when the subscapularis muscle had to be repaired via an anterior approach or the infraspinatus muscle via a posterior approach from the proximal humerus attachment point, following release. In such patients, the time of immobilization is extended to 6 weeks [47, 57]. After 4–6 weeks, the sling is removed, followed by active-assisted or active full range of motion in all planes [1]. Progressive resistance training is initiated during the 6–8 week postoperative period [58]. Full return to activities and noncontact sports is permitted at 3–4 months postoperatively, based on individual tolerance and recovery progress [1]. Additionally, recent studies are exploring new rehabilitation techniques and devices, such as wearable sensors to monitor scapular motion, which can more accurately assess patients' rehabilitation progress and offer personalized training guidance [59].

Scapular glenoid fractures present significant clinical challenges, with both operative and nonoperative management strategies carrying substantial risks of complications and suboptimal outcomes. Conservative treatment frequently results in unfavorable long-term sequelae, including chronic pain, dysfunction, shoulder instability, and post-traumatic osteoarthritis [27, 60]. Complications associated with operative management of glenoid fractures include (but not limited to): (1) infection, shoulder stiffness, (2) rotator cuff weakness (due to retraction or tenotomy), (3) problems related to hardware, (4) nerve injury, and (5) heterotopic ossification.

Seiornandez et al. documented 93 complications in operatively and nonoperatively managed scapular fractures. Among surgically treated cases, the most frequent complications were painful hardware requiring removal (11 cases), stiffness requiring manipulation under anesthesia (6 cases), and heterotopic ossification (7 cases) [27]. Anavian et al., in a study of 33 patients with intra-articularly displaced glenoid fractures, found that one patient had articular screw placement, one had postoperative stiffness, and one underwent surgical resection of asymptomatic heterotopic bone around the glenoid joint [61]. Of particular concern, a study found that 39% of patients (10 cases) exhibited postoperative subscapularis insufficiency, mainly presenting with limited shoulder internal rotation [62]. Although nerve injuries often accompany glenoid fractures, it can be challenging to determine whether palsies, such as axillary, brachial plexus, or suprascapular nerve palsies, are caused by the initial trauma or subsequent surgical intervention. Therefore, a thorough preoperative nerve evaluation is essential. A systematic retrospective analysis of 2560 Latarjet procedures revealed an overall complication rate of 16.1%, with nerve injuries (including axillary, musculocutaneous, and suprascapular nerve injuries, among others) occurring at a rate of 1.9% [63].

8. Conclusions

Glenoid fractures, though uncommon, pose a challenge to the orthopedic surgeon and come with a range of surgical treatment options. Glenoid fractures are often associated with shoulder dislocation, injuries to the SSSC, clavicle fractures, humerus fractures, rib fractures, and chest injuries. Therefore, it is crucial to pay attention to differential diagnosis. We have summarized the available evidence on treatment algorithms for different types of glenoid fractures. A variety of surgical approaches, including open repositioning and internal fixation techniques as well as arthroscopic repair and assisted fixation techniques, have been described and have yielded encouraging results. Moreover, it is anticipated that the use of surgical treatment may increase in the future, driven by advancements in arthroscopic, robotic, and navigational fixation techniques.

Conflict of interest

The authors declare no conflict of interest.

Notes/thanks/other declarations

We gratefully acknowledge the valuable contributions of Professor Yan Xiong from the Second Affiliated Hospital of Zhejiang University School of Medicine and Dr. Xiang Zheng, attending orthopedic surgeon at Lishui Central Hospital. The authors would also like to thank our department colleagues, the hospital, and the patients for their dedication.

Author details

Shuming Huang*, Shuhua Lan, Panpan Xie and Jiekai Ye
Department of Orthopaedic Surgery, The Fifth Affiliated Hospital of Wenzhou Medical University; Lishui Municipal Central Hospital, Lishui, Zhejiang, China

*Address all correspondence to: smhuang001@163.com

References

[1] Seidl AJ, Joyce CD. Acute fractures of the glenoid. Journal of the American Academy of Orthopaedic Surgeons. 2020;**28**(22):e978-e987. DOI: 10.5435/jaaos-d-20-00252

[2] Ström P. Glenoid fractures of the shoulder. EFORT Open Reviews. 2020;**5**(10):620-623. DOI: 10.1302/2058-5241.5.190057

[3] Wu D, Zhang G, Zhou Z, Song W, Chen D, Bai Z, et al. Arthroscopic suture anchor fixation results in similar clinical outcomes, less range of motion limitation, but poorer quality of reduction compared to open screw fixation for acute large anterior glenoid rim fractures. Journal of Shoulder and Elbow Surgery. 2025;**34**(4):944-954. DOI: 10.1016/j.jse.2024.07.013

[4] Tatro JM, Schroder LK, Molitor BA, Parker ED, Cole PA. Injury mechanism, epidemiology, and hospital trends of scapula fractures: A 10-year retrospective study of the National Trauma Data Bank. Injury. 2019;**50**(2):376-381. DOI: 10.1016/j.injury.2019.01.017

[5] Vander Voort W, Wilkinson B, Bedard N, Hendrickson N, Willey M. The operative treatment of scapula fractures: An analysis of 10,097 patients. The Iowa Orthopaedic Journal. 2022;**42**(1):213-216

[6] Schmidt V, Mukka S, Bergdahl C, Ekholm C, Bruggemann A, Wolf O. Epidemiology, treatment, and mortality of 3973 scapula fractures from the Swedish fracture register. Journal of Shoulder and Elbow Surgery. 2025;**34**(1):e47-e56. DOI: 10.1016/j.jse.2024.03.024

[7] Frich LH, Larsen MS. How to deal with a glenoid fracture. EFORT Open Reviews. 2017;**2**(5):151-157. DOI: 10.1302/2058-5241.2.160082

[8] Launonen AP, Laitinen MK, Sumrein BO, Niemi ST, Kannus P, Mattila VM. Trends in scapular fractures: A nationwide 17-year study in Finland. JSES International. 2020;**4**(1):59-62. DOI: 10.1016/j.jses.2019.10.111

[9] Mavrotas J, Fischer J. Scapula fractures: Functional anatomy, clinical assessment and management. British Journal of Hospital Medicine (London, England). 2024;**85**(3):1-8. DOI: 10.12968/hmed.2023.0351

[10] Almajed YA, Hall AC, Gillingwater TH, Alashkham A. Anatomical, functional and biomechanical review of the glenoid labrum. Journal of Anatomy. 2022;**240**(4):761-771. DOI: 10.1111/joa.13582

[11] Soslowsky LJ, Flatow EL, Bigliani LU, Mow VC. Articular geometry of the glenohumeral joint. Clinical Orthopaedics and Related Research. 1992;**285**:181-190

[12] Rayes J, Xu J, Sparavalo S, Ma J, Jonah L, Wong I. Calculating glenoid bone loss based on glenoid height using ipsilateral three-dimensional computed tomography. Knee Surgery, Sports Traumatology, Arthroscopy. 2023;**31**(1):169-176. DOI: 10.1007/s00167-022-07020-4

[13] Tankala M, Senapati S, Behera SS, Shamal S. The glenoid Fossa's morphometric investigation and its clinical implications. Cureus. 2023;**15**(6):e39981. DOI: 10.7759/cureus.39981

[14] Piponov HI, Savin D, Shah N, Esposito D, Schwartz B, Moretti V, et al. Glenoid version and size: Does gender, ethnicity, or body size play a role? International Orthopaedics. 2016;**40**(11):2347-2353. DOI: 10.1007/s00264-016-3201-8

[15] Johnson CM, DeFoor MT, Griswold BG, Bozzone AE, Galvin JW, Parada SA. Functional anatomy and biomechanics of shoulder instability. Clinics in Sports Medicine. 2024;**43**(4):547-565. DOI: 10.1016/j.csm.2024.03.016

[16] Limb D. Scapula fractures: A review. EFORT Open Reviews. 2021;**6**(6):518-525. DOI: 10.1302/2058-5241.6.210010

[17] Berritto D, Pinto A, Russo A, Urraro F, Laporta A, Belfiore MP, et al. Scapular fractures: a common diagnostic pitfall. Acta Bio-Medica. 2018;**89**(1-S):102-110. DOI: 10.23750/abm.v89i1-S.7014

[18] Ropp AM, Davis DL. Scapular fractures: What radiologists need to know. AJR. American Journal of Roentgenology. 2015;**205**(3):491-501. DOI: 10.2214/AJR.15.14446

[19] Ross KJ, Tomkinson GR, McGregor BF, Ayres OC, Piscitelli D. Addition of the apical oblique projection increases the detection of acute traumatic shoulder abnormalities in adults. Emergency Radiology. 2017;**24**(4):329-334. DOI: 10.1007/s10140-017-1483-9

[20] Yimam HM, Dey R, Rachuene PA, Kauta NJ, Roche SJL, Sivarasu S. Identification of recurring scapular fracture patterns using 3-dimensional computerized fracture mapping. Journal of Shoulder and Elbow Surgery. 2022;**31**(3):571-579. DOI: 10.1016/j.jse.2021.08.036

[21] Vosshenrich J, Bruno M, Cantarelli Rodrigues T, Donners R, Jardon M, Leonhardt Y, et al. Arthroscopy-validated diagnostic performance of 7-minute five-sequence deep learning super-resolution 3-T shoulder MRI. Radiology. 2025;**314**(2):e241351. DOI: 10.1148/radiol.241351

[22] Goss TP. Fractures of the glenoid cavity. The Journal of Bone and Joint Surgery. American Volume. 1992;**74**(2):299-305

[23] Ideberg R, Grevsten S, Larsson S. Epidemiology of scapular fractures. Incidence and classification of 338 fractures. Acta Orthopaedica Scandinavica. 1995;**66**(5):395-397. DOI: 10.3109/17453679508995571

[24] Meinberg EG, Agel J, Roberts CS, Karam MD, Kellam JF. Fracture and dislocation classification Compendium-2018. Journal of Orthopaedic Trauma. 2018;**32**(Suppl. 1):S1-S170. DOI: 10.1097/BOT.0000000000001063

[25] Bartonicek J, Tucek M, Klika D, Chochola A. Pathoanatomy and computed tomography classification of glenoid fossa fractures based on ninety patients. International Orthopaedics. 2016;**40**(11):2383-2392. DOI: 10.1007/s00264-016-3169-4

[26] Gilbert F, Eden L, Meffert R, Konietschke F, Lotz J, Bauer L, et al. Intra- and interobserver reliability of glenoid fracture classifications by Ideberg, Euler and AO. BMC Musculoskeletal Disorders. 2018;**19**(1):89. DOI: 10.1186/s12891-018-2016-8

[27] Sernandez HC, Riehl JT, Fogel J. Sling and forget it? A systematic review of operative versus nonoperative outcomes for scapula fractures. Journal of Shoulder

and Elbow Surgery. 2024;**33**(12):2743-2754. DOI: 10.1016/j.jse.2024.05.042

[28] Bi AS, Kane LT, Butler BA, Stover MD. Outcomes following extra-articular fractures of the scapula: A systematic review. Injury. 2020;**51**(3):602-610. DOI: 10.1016/j.injury.2020.01.036

[29] Willms S, Caines A, Buckley R. Is it true that most intra-articular glenoid fractures should have surgery? Injury. 2024;**55**(11):111880. DOI: 10.1016/j.injury.2024.111880

[30] van Oostveen DP, Temmerman OP, Burger BJ, van Noort A, Robinson M. Glenoid fractures: A review of pathology, classification, treatment and results. Acta Orthopaedica Belgica. 2014;**80**(1):88-98

[31] Wieser K, Waltenspul M, Ernstbrunner L, Ammann E, Nieuwland A, Eid K, et al. Nonoperative treatment of anterior glenoid rim fractures after first-time traumatic anterior shoulder dislocation: A study with 9-year follow-up. Journal of Bone and Joint Surgery Open Access. 2020;**5**(4):e20.00133. DOI: 10.2106/JBJS.OA.20.00133

[32] Cole PA, Freeman G, Dubin JR. Scapula fractures. Current Reviews in Musculoskeletal Medicine. 2013;**6**(1):79-87. DOI: 10.1007/s12178-012-9151-x

[33] Dickens JF, Slaven SE, Cameron KL, Pickett AM, Posner M, Campbell SE, et al. Prospective evaluation of glenoid bone loss after first-time and recurrent anterior glenohumeral instability events. The American Journal of Sports Medicine. 2019;**47**(5):1082-1089. DOI: 10.1177/0363546519831286

[34] Weisberg Z, Cole W, Rumps MV, Vopat B, Mulcahey MK. Bony Bankart lesion: Diagnosis, management, and outcomes. JBJS Reviews. 2024;**12**(5):e23.00200. DOI: 10.2106/JBJS.RVW.23.00200

[35] Secci G, Lazzarini F, Distefano M, Porciatti T, Tonelli F, Mugnaini M, et al. Impact of size and fragmentation of the anteroinferior glenoid rim on clinical and functional outcomes of non-operatively treated bony Bankart lesions in middle-aged population. Archives of Orthopaedic and Trauma Surgery. 2024;**144**(8):3533-3539. DOI: 10.1007/s00402-024-05466-4

[36] Ding H, Bao Y-G, Yin B, Chang Q-H, Zai Q-S, Shi Q, et al. Efficacy analysis of axillary approach in the treatment of Ideberg type I and II scapular glenoid fractures: Case series. Medicine. 2023;**102**(28):e34333. DOI: 10.1097/md.0000000000034333

[37] Li B, Rong K, Deng H, Tang Z, Tang J, Sun J. Double-pulley, V-shaped fixation technique for arthroscopic repair of ideberg type IA glenoid fracture. Journal of Orthopaedic Surgery (Hong Kong). 2024;**32**(2):10225536241254913. DOI: 10.1177/10225536241254913

[38] Boehm E, Keck A, Krueger D, Scheibel M. Arthroscopic repair of anteroinferior glenoid rim fractures: Mean 10-year clinical and radiologic results. Journal of Shoulder and Elbow Surgery. 2024;**33**(12):2893-2898. DOI: 10.1016/j.jse.2024.07.027

[39] Park I, Shin SJ. Arthroscopic double-row bridge fixation provided satisfactory shoulder functional restoration with high union rate for acute anterior glenoid fracture. Knee Surgery, Sports Traumatology, Arthroscopy. 2023;**31**(7):2681-2687. DOI: 10.1007/s00167-023-07389-w

[40] Scheibel M, Hug K, Gerhardt C, Krueger D. Arthroscopic reduction

and fixation of large solitary and multifragmented anterior glenoid rim fractures. Journal of Shoulder and Elbow Surgery. 2016;**25**(5):781-790. DOI: 10.1016/j.jse.2015.09.012

[41] Mousa H, Aresti N. Arthroscopic reduction internal fixation for glenoid fractures: A systematic review of the outcomes and complications. Musculoskeletal Surgery. 2025;**109**(2):127-132. DOI: 10.1007/s12306-024-00870-w

[42] Tao MA, Garrigues GE. Arthroscopic-assisted fixation of Ideberg type III glenoid fractures. Arthroscopy Techniques. 2015;**4**(2):e119-e125. DOI: 10.1016/j.eats.2014.11.012

[43] Lin IH, Lin T-L, Chang H-W, Lin C-Y, Tsai C-H, Lo C-S, et al. Arthroscopy-assisted reduction and internal fixation versus open reduction and internal fixation for glenoid fracture with scapular involvement: A retrospective cohort study. Journal of Clinical Medicine. 2022;**11**(4):1131. DOI: 10.3390/jcm11041131

[44] Taverna E, Guarrella V, Freehill MT, Garavaglia G. Arthroscopic reduction with endobutton fixation for glenoid fracture. Joints. 2017;**5**(2):127-130. DOI: 10.1055/s-0037-1603675

[45] Morash K, Ravipati APT, Wong IH. Arthroscopic, nonrigid fixation of a displaced glenoid fracture after anterior shoulder dislocation. Arthroscopy Techniques. 2020;**9**(2):e233-e237. DOI: 10.1016/j.eats.2019.10.001

[46] Zhang X, Jiang Z, Chu FL, Jia DL, Han XG, Li XY, et al. Comparative study of trans-axillary approach and Delto-pectoral approach to the treatment of Ideberg types I and II scapular glenoid fractures. Orthopaedic Surgery. 2025;**17**(5):1349-1358. DOI: 10.1111/os.70012

[47] Pfister G, Murison JC, Sabate-Ferris A, Danis J, De l'Escalopier N, Mathieu L. Open screw fixation of large anterior glenoid rim fractures using a Deltopectoral approach with subscapularis splitting. Techniques in Hand & Upper Extremity Surgery. 2022;**26**(3):188-192. DOI: 10.1097/BTH.0000000000000383

[48] Altun G, Shatat K, Kapicioglu M, Ersen A, Bilsel K. Surgical treatment of scapula body fractures extending glenoid fossa: Surgical technique and early results. Turkish Journal of Trauma and Emergency Surgery. 2022;**28**(10):1508-1513. DOI: 10.14744/tjtes.2022.27715

[49] Lim EJ, Jeong H-S, Kim K-J. Posterior deltoid-sparing approach for displaced inferior or posterior glenoid fossa fractures: Technical note and case series. Scientific Reports. 2024;**14**(1):6500. DOI: 10.1038/s41598-024-56974-7

[50] Obremskey WT, Lyman JR. A modified judet approach to the scapula. Journal of Orthopaedic Trauma. 2004;**18**(10):696-699. DOI: 10.1097/00005131-200411000-00007

[51] Wang H, Lin J-r, Wei G-z, Wu G, Qiu Y-Y, Xie Y. A clinical study on the effect of axillary approach in the treatment of Ideberg type II scapular glenoid fractures. BMC Surgery. 2024;**24**(1):319. DOI: 10.1186/s12893-024-02623-9

[52] Hong NW, Jones CW, Hong TF. Deltoid takedown approach to Ideberg VI/AO F2(4) glenoid fossa fractures. JSES Reviews, Reports, and Techniques. 2022;**2**(4):559-570. DOI: 10.1016/j.xrrt.2022.06.005

[53] Shen C, Dong J, Xu M, Zhang J, Li X. Superior approach to the glenoid for

treating acromion fractures combined with ideberg type III scapular glenoid fractures: A technical note. International Orthopaedics. 2024;**48**(10):2749-2754. DOI: 10.1007/s00264-024-06273-7

[54] Maier D, Izadpanah K, Ogon P, Mutzel M, Bayer J, Sudkamp NP, et al. Open fixation of acute anterior glenoid rim fractures with bioresorbable pins: Analysis of clinical and radiological outcome. Archives of Orthopaedic and Trauma Surgery. 2015;**135**(7):953-961. DOI: 10.1007/s00402-015-2242-6

[55] Lou W, Chen J, Li M, Xu D. A new surgical approach for the treatment of scapular glenoid fractures- axillary approach: A single center case series. Annals of Medicine & Surgery. 2022;**79**:104029. DOI: 10.1016/j.amsu.2022.104029

[56] Dobelle E, Robert S, Gaujac N, Laumonerie P, Mansat P, Bonnevialle N. Scapular fractures osteosynthesis via Judet's posterior approach: Clinical and radiographic results. International Orthopaedics. 2023;**47**(6):1557-1564. DOI: 10.1007/s00264-023-05754-5

[57] Jenssen KK, Lundgreen K, Madsen JE, Kvakestad R, Pripp AH, Dimmen S. No functional difference between three and six weeks of immobilization after arthroscopic rotator cuff repair: A prospective randomized controlled non-inferiority trial. Arthroscopy. 2018;**34**(10):2765-2774. DOI: 10.1016/j.arthro.2018.05.036

[58] Hinz M, Kruckeberg BM, Davis CS, Cinque ME, Horan MP, Drumm A, et al. Minimum 10-year clinical and functional outcomes after arthroscopic bony Bankart bridge for the treatment of bony Bankart lesions. Journal of Shoulder and Elbow Surgery. 2025;**34**(6S):S57-S63. DOI: 10.1016/j.jse.2025.02.002

[59] Sun JN, Zheng QY, Wang RS, Ma YR, Chen P. An additional rehabilitation program to improve postoperative outcomes in patients with rotator cuff tear and scapular dyskinesis: A propensity score-matched study. BMC Musculoskeletal Disorders. 2025;**26**(1):338. DOI: 10.1186/s12891-025-08596-x

[60] Konigshausen M, Patzholz S, Coulibaly M, Nicolas V, Vandemeulebroecke M, Schildhauer TA, et al. Instability and results after non-operative treatment of large anterior glenoid rim fractures: Is there a correlation between fragment size or displacement and recurrence? Archives of Orthopaedic and Trauma Surgery. 2022;**142**(10):2727-2738. DOI: 10.1007/s00402-021-04020-w

[61] Anavian J, Gauger EM, Schroder LK, Wijdicks CA, Cole PA. Surgical and functional outcomes after operative management of complex and displaced intra-articular glenoid fractures. The Journal of Bone and Joint Surgery. American Volume. 2012;**94**(7):645-653. DOI: 10.2106/JBJS.J.00896

[62] Maier D, Izadpanah K, Bayer J, Langenmair ER, Ogon P, Sudkamp NP, et al. Influencing factors and complications in open treatment of acute anterior glenoid rim fractures. Der Unfallchirurg. 2017;**120**(4):320-328. DOI: 10.1007/s00113-015-0129-1

[63] Cho C-H, Na SS, Choi B-C, Kim D-H. Complications related to Latarjet shoulder stabilization: A systematic review. The American Journal of Sports Medicine. 2021;**51**(1):263-270. DOI: 10.1177/03635465211042314

Section 3

Complex and Chronic Conditions

Chapter 5

Revitalizing Shoulder Wellness: Innovative Approaches to Rehabilitation for Rotator Cuff Injuries

Emine Merve Ersever

Abstract

The shoulder joint is the body part with a complex anatomy and the widest range of motion compared to other joints. Rotator cuff problems are the most common cause of shoulder pain. Seventy-four percent of rotator cuff dysfunctions cause severe shoulder pain. The decrease in the quality of daily living activities causes significant joint limitations and injuries. Decreased nutrition of the rotator cuff tendons can result from internal factors like microstructural collagen abnormalities, variations in fiber properties, the shape of the coracoacromial arch, genetic influences, and hormonal changes. External factors include stress overload, kinematic irregularities, and repetitive use. Rehabilitation for rotator cuff tears focuses on pain management, improving range of motion, maintaining scapulothoracic rhythm, and restoring functionality. Treatment of rotator cuff tendinopathy injuries yields successful results with many conservative options (including exercise, electrotherapy, acupuncture, manual therapy, injection therapy, and taping). In shoulder rehabilitation, the primary focus should be on the elimination of pain and the restoration of functional movements through dynamic stability of the rotator cuff and scapular muscles. Neuromuscular re-education is provided, especially with therapeutic exercises, and the aim is to strengthen the shoulder girdle muscles and achieve an adequate range of motion.

Keywords: rotator cuff tendinopathies, shoulder rehabilitation, shoulder exercises, shoulder stability

1. Introduction

The journey towards restoring shoulder health for individuals suffering from rotator cuff injuries demands a comprehensive understanding of innovative rehabilitation methods. Modern approaches to recovery go beyond traditional techniques, incorporating advancements in physical therapy, targeted exercises, and technology-driven interventions.

A critical element of these innovative rehabilitation strategies is the emphasis on tailored exercise regimens. These programs are designed to strengthen the muscles surrounding the shoulder joint, enhancing stability and improving range of motion. For instance, resistance band exercises and rotator cuff-focused strength training not only help in rebuilding muscle but also aid in pain management and functional recovery. Additionally, the integration of modalities such as ultrasound therapy, electrical stimulation, and cryotherapy has been shown to accelerate healing processes by reducing inflammation and promoting tissue regeneration. Nutrition also plays a pivotal role in shoulder recovery; a diet rich in anti-inflammatory foods and essential nutrients supports optimal healing and overall wellness.Furthermore, incorporating technology through wearable devices can provide real-time feedback on movement patterns, helping practitioners fine-tune rehabilitation strategies. This personalized approach ensures that rehabilitation plans are closely monitored and adapted to each patient's unique needs and progress.

The four muscles, collectively known as the rotator cuff muscles, form a protective sheath (or cuff) around the shoulder joint, comprising the tendons of the supraspinatus, infraspinatus, subscapularis, and teres minor [1]. These muscles originate from the body of the scapula and attach to the tuberosity of the proximal humerus. The rotator cuff muscles play a crucial role in stabilizing the glenohumeral joint, particularly during abduction. Their primary function is to ensure the dynamic stability of the GH joint by compressing the humeral head against the glenoid. This compression helps to resist glenohumeral movement and control rotations across all planes, keeping the humeral head centered within the glenoid [2]. For all this to happen, four muscles must work in synchrony. Eccentric and concentric contraction of the rotator cuff muscles plays a primary role in providing dynamic stabilization during movement. They are also responsible for force absorption and compression between joint surfaces.

In general, tendinopathies are prevalent "overuse" injuries characterized by load-related pain and a reduction in function. A 2019 symposium on tendinopathies regarded the terms "subacromial pain syndrome" (or impingement) and "rotator cuff-related shoulder pain" as synonyms, both referring to pain associated with the shoulder tendons and the consequent loss of function [3]. The symptoms of this condition typically include minimal pain at rest, a largely preserved range of motion, and heightened pain during resistance training. Evidence indicates that the disability resulting from rotator cuff tendinopathy significantly affects daily life, leading to social burdens such as absenteeism and increased healthcare costs. Approximately half of those affected experience these issues for over 12 continuous months and often resort to surgery as a solution [3, 4].

Research on the architectural characteristics of rotator cuff muscles indicates that these four muscles are primarily optimized for force production, aligning with their function as stabilizers of the shoulder. Even minor alterations in muscle architecture can significantly impact shoulder function. Therefore, a comprehensive understanding of the muscular structure of these four muscles is invaluable for shoulder rehabilitation and treatment [5]. The type of muscle fibers, whether fusiform or pennate, significantly impacts muscle strength. Pennate muscles, characterized by the presence of intramuscular tendons, are considerably stronger than their fusiform counterparts. The supraspinatus, infraspinatus, and teres minor are examples of pennate muscles, each containing intramuscular tendons [6]. The subscapularis is classified as a multipennate muscle featuring 4–6 intramuscular tendons, and it is anatomically challenging to identify its extramural tendons. Additionally, there are three distinct facets on the tuberculum majus: the upper, middle, and lower facets. The supraspinatus muscle attaches to the upper and slightly middle facets, while the infraspinatus and teres minor muscles connect to the lower facet. The focus has been on the supraspinatus muscle due to its important role in rotator cuff tendinopathies. Regardless of the cause, other than acute trauma, the first pathological change that disrupts the normal structure in the RC is tendinopathy [7]. This change is most commonly seen in the supraspinatus tendon. This region, characterized by inadequate vascularization, is believed to be the primary factor contributing to supraspinatus tendonitis. The supraspinatus muscle's limited blood supply leads to increased fatigue during overhead activities due to heightened intramuscular pressure. Additionally, the hypovascularization impedes the migration of macrophages, mast cells, and T cells—key cells involved in tendon repair—to the damaged area, rendering the supraspinatus muscle more susceptible to injury [5–7].

2. Physiological mechanisms underlying rotator cuff injuries

Although various theories have been proposed to explain the physiological basis of rotator cuff tendinopathies (RCT), some underlying mechanisms remain poorly understood and warrant further study. The existing literature generally classifies the causes of these tendon disorders into two main groups: intrinsic factors, which include age-related degeneration and microscopic tendon tears, and extrinsic factors, which involve biomechanical stresses and external pressures that can lead to tendon irritation and injury [8, 9]. This classification emphasizes the complex and multifactorial nature of rotator cuff dysfunction and highlights the need for thorough research to fully elucidate the intricate interactions among these contributing factors (see **Tables 1** and **2**).

Extrinsic factors are divided into two subgroups: primary and secondary [10].

Primary subacromial impingement is frequently seen in young populations, especially in athletes, as a result of abnormal mechanical relationships between the RK and the coracoacromial arch. Neer divided primary subacromial impingement into three stages [11].

Stage 1: Edema and inflammation.

Stage 2: Fibrosis and tendonitis.

Stage 3: Bone spurs and tendon ruptures.

Intrinsic factors
Mechanical collagen stretching
Matrix component damage
Changes in vascularity
Metabolic changes
Overuse of tendons
Anatomical or bone anomalies
Hyaline, mucoid, and myxoid-type degenerations

Table 1.
Intrinsic factors contributing to rotator cuff tendinopathy.

Extrinsic factors
Muscle imbalance
Motor control problems
Disruption of functional arc of movement
Postural change
Training errors
Occupational or environmental risk
Extrinsic factors are divided into two subgroups: primary and secondary

Table 2.
Extrinsic factors contributing to rotator cuff tendinopathy.

Secondary subacromial impingement occurs when there is a relative narrowing of the subacromial space, primarily due to excessive demands on the rotator cuff to provide dynamic stabilization of the shoulder. This can arise from factors such as glenohumeral hypermobility, scapular dyskinesia, tension in the posterior capsule, muscle weakness, and fatigue [12]. During arm movements, compression of the rotator cuff muscles within the subacromial space may lead to degeneration, particularly of the supraspinatus tendon, resulting in structural deterioration. Prolonged and repetitive compression can give rise to microtears and potentially partial or full-thickness tears of the tendon. These repetitive micro-traumas can trigger acute inflammation in the synovial tissue, resulting in pain and functional impairment due to an increase in pro-inflammatory cytokines within the synovium [11, 12].

The study by Clark and Harryman on rotator cuff tendons, capsules, and ligaments also classified microscopically the RK muscle pathologies into five layers [13].

Layer 1: This layer is situated adjacent to the obliquely oriented KH ligament fibers, corresponding to each muscle axis. Arterioles are broadly distributed throughout this layer.

Layer 2: Composed of parallel tendon fibers that are organized into large, tightly packed bundles, this layer contains arterioles nestled between the crossing fascicles.

Layer 3: This layer features fascicles that are smaller than those in Layer 2 and are not as densely packed. Blood vessels, although present, are smaller compared to those in the previous layer.

Layer 4: Characterized by thin, ribbon-like collagen fibers, this layer consists of loose connective tissue. Here, only blood vessels and capillaries are present, located adjacent to the extra-articular surface of the shoulder capsule.

Layer 5: This thin layer adheres to the humerus through delicately woven collagen fibrils, resembling Sharpey's fibers found in bone.

3. Clinical evaluation

3.1 Pain

Pain is often the most common symptom associated with shoulder pathologies. It is crucial to assess the pain experienced during rest, activity, and at night, as this can provide valuable insight into the underlying condition and guide the appropriate physiotherapy approach. For instance, if a patient experiences pain at night, it typically indicates inflammation, and treatment modalities that might exacerbate inflammation should be avoided. Rest pain can be evaluated similarly; however, if the pain occurs only during activity, it is likely related to a mechanical issue. In such cases, it is important to examine how normal movement biomechanics are affected and identify the source of the abnormal movement [14].

3.2 Range of motion

Assessing joint movement is a crucial aspect of differential diagnosis for various pathologies. When evaluating joint movement, it is essential to examine painless active joint movement, along with both active and passive joint movements. In cases of impingement syndrome, a reduction in joint mobility is typically observed due to pain; however, passive joint movement remains unaffected. In contrast, the key distinguishing feature of a frozen shoulder is the restriction of passive joint movement. Conditions such as impingement syndrome, rotator cuff tears, or humeral issues should be considered in this context. However, in terms of evaluating functionality, it is important to remember to evaluate active total elevation and active internal rotation [15].

3.3 Muscle strength

Assessing the strength of muscles within the painful range provides highly reliable information. If muscle strength is preserved during the test, it may lead to an underestimation of the normal strength values. After pain has diminished, evaluating muscle strength becomes crucial for identifying any imbalances and devising an appropriate exercise program [16].

3.4 Evaluation of scapular movement

Evaluation of scapular movements is important in determining the exercises to be given. In the clinic, scapular movement can be evaluated observationally and with the lateral scapular slide (Kibler) test [17]. In the laboratory environment, three-dimensional analysis systems provide the opportunity for objective measurement in the evaluation of scapular movement. However, since these systems are expensive and the evaluations take a long time, they are mostly used in scientific studies. Although the lateral scapular slide test can be easily applied in the clinic, different results have been reported regarding its reliability [17, 18]. It can be preferred, especially in unilateral scapular dyskinesia, in order to give an idea. The test is performed in three different positions. In the first position, the patient is standing, the arms are at the side of the body, and the distance between the inferior angle of the scapula and the collumna vertebralis is measured with a tape measure. In the second position, with the arms on the waist, and in the third position, with the arm in 90-degree abduction and internal rotation, the distance between the inferior angle of the scapula and the vertebrae collumna is evaluated and compared with the healthy side.

3.5 Palpation

It is important to evaluate the tenderness of soft tissues. Especially the evaluation of the tenderness of the rotator cuff muscles, the long head of the biceps brachii, the pectoralis minor, and the posterior capsule by palpation is important for the manual therapy methods to be applied [19].

3.6 Functional activity level

How well patients return to their daily activities is actually one of the most important determinants of the success of the treatment. Different questionnaires are used for this. The most commonly used ones are DASH-T, ASES questionnaire, Constant-Murley questionnaire, SPADI, etc. [20].

4. Treatment approaches in rotator cuff tendinopathy

In treating RCT injuries, conservative methods are usually the first choice. Surgical intervention is considered when conservative treatment does not provide sufficient relief. The primary goals of RCT treatment should be to alleviate pain and restore functional movements while ensuring dynamic stabilization of the rotator cuff and scapular muscles. The processes of tissue repair and inflammation play a crucial role in determining the pace and objectives of both treatment and exercise progression. These processes guide therapists in deciding whether to adopt a more aggressive approach or to exercise caution, particularly in cases of an irritable shoulder where pain management is prioritized. During rehabilitation, it is essential to find a balance between restoring shoulder mobility and allowing for the healing of soft tissues [20–23].

4.1 Conservative treatment

Conservative treatment of RCT includes pharmacological treatments, exercises, electrotherapy, and patient education programs.

4.2 Pharmacological treatment

Pharmacological approaches for treating RKL can be administered orally, topically, or through intra-articular injection. Oral medications include paracetamol, non-steroidal anti-inflammatory drugs (NSAIDs), opioid analgesics, and psychotropic medications. Additionally, NSAIDs may be applied topically to the skin. In recent years, intra-articular injection has become a frequently utilized treatment method.

Corticosteroids, hyaluronic acid, or platelet-enriched plasma are administered in the glenohumeral or subacromial space [24]. This approach is commonly favored due to its practical application, minimal systemic side effects, and rapid pain relief. However, the long-term outcomes and overall effectiveness of these treatments have not been definitively established in the existing literature [14].

4.3 Thermal agents and manual applications

Thermal agents encompass superficial heat agents, cryotherapy (cold therapy), and deep heat applications. Thermotherapy involves the use of hot or cold treatments to alter the temperature of soft tissues, skin, and joints. These thermal agents play a significant role in managing pain, tissue metabolism, edema, and inflammation by influencing blood circulation and the chemical reactions occurring within the body. Additionally, they help regulate mechanical modalities, as well as intracellular and intercellular fluid balances [25].

Cold therapy reduces blood flow by inducing vasoconstriction and lowering the temperature of skin and soft tissues. This leads to a decrease in nerve conduction speed, inflammation, and metabolic rate. When tissue and joint temperatures fall to 30°C or below, it inhibits enzymes such as collagenase, elastase, and hyaluronidase, resulting in cellular hypoxia, which helps reduce edema and the presence of inflammatory mediators. The use of cold affects the exchanges between Ca^{2+} and Na^{+}, causing opposite irritation, thus increasing pain tolerance. In the literature, ice application is recommended as an effective treatment for cryotherapy. The application time varies between 10 and 30 min. Cutaneous changes occur within 6–12 min. It can be in the form of ice massage, cold packs, sprays, and ice immersion [26].

Among the various superficial heat applications, hot packs and paraffin are the most commonly used agents, typically offering a maximum penetration depth of 1 cm or less. The recommended duration for both treatments is 20 minutes. In terms of deep heating modalities, ultrasound (US) is the most widely utilized therapeutic agent. The frequency setting for ultrasound is adjusted based on the depth of the tissue being treated. Higher frequencies result in energy absorption primarily in superficial tissues, while lower frequencies allow for deeper tissue penetration and absorption. Specifically, 1 MHz ultrasound is effective for treating tissues located 3–7 cm deep, such as the rotator cuff, gastrocnemius, and vastus intermedius muscles. Conversely, 3 MHz ultrasound is better suited for treating tissues that are more than 3 cm superficial, including the patellar tendon, medial collateral ligament, and brachialis muscle [27].

Manual therapies, including deep tissue massage, joint mobilization, trigger point release techniques, transverse friction massage, soft tissue mobilization, visceral mobilization, and proprioceptive neuromuscular facilitation, involve passive movements that are applied gently and slowly, often incorporating oscillations. Additionally, the definition provided by orthopedic manual therapy professionals encompasses pain modulation, neural tissue mobility, movement control, muscle stabilization, and the enhancement of functional capabilities [28].

Deep friction techniques and deep tissue massages, which are part of manual therapy approaches, induce traumatic hyperemia in the tissues and stimulate both Type I and II mechanoreceptors. The afferent impulses generated from the moved structures override pain stimuli, resulting in temporary analgesia. Furthermore, deep transverse friction massage promotes the shortening of collagen tissue and regulates interstitial fluid content, leading to improved mobility. It is advisable to administer manual treatments for a duration of at least 4 weeks, three times a week, for 10–20 minutes each session [28, 29].

5. Rehabilitation and exercise strategies

Several individual factors, including the patient's age, expectations, activity level, tear size, as well as any atrophy and degenerative changes present, influence the selection of treatment. During the acute phase, early rehabilitation prioritizes addressing pain, inflammation, and edema while restoring the normal range of motion. Preferred interventions include ice application, electrical stimulation, laser therapy, manual therapy, dry needling, low-dose intermittent ultrasound, pendulum exercises, and isometric exercises. The objectives of early rehabilitation encompass reducing muscle inhibition, preserving the integrity of the repair with a tear, and promoting independence in modified movements.

Immobilization during the initial 3–5 days of the acute phase facilitates the progression of both the inflammation and proliferation phases. Supporting the shoulder at a 45° angle in abduction, with the elbow flexed at 90° and the shoulder in internal rotation, enhances blood flow to the supraspinatus. This positioning also alleviates tension on the tendon caused by reflexive muscle contractions within the supraspinatus [30]. Additionally, Grade 1–2 joint mobilization and passive joint movements are beneficial in promoting the formation of regular collagen fibers, fostering muscle relaxation, and preventing the development of adhesions (**Figure 1**) [31].

The goal of rehabilitation during the subacute middle phase is to facilitate soft tissue healing while avoiding excessive tension on the recovering tissues and ensuring optimal neuromuscular control. Early mobilization plays a crucial role in influencing both longitudinal and transverse displacement of tissues and tendons, as well as enhancing tensile strength. Mobilization techniques can be particularly beneficial during the early fibroplasia stage due to the reformation of collagen tissue (**Figure 2**).

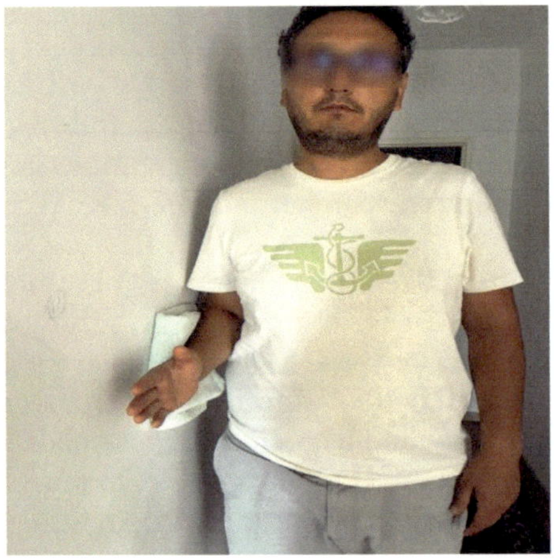

Figure 1.
Isometric shoulder external rotation.

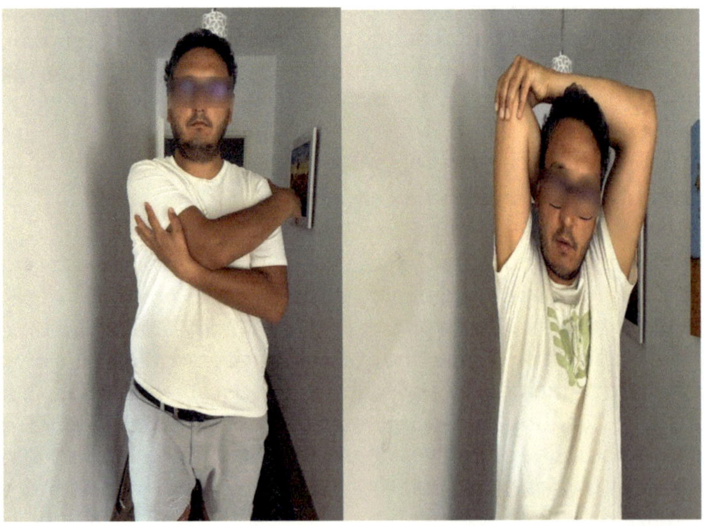

Figure 2.
Posterior capsule stretching.

Research indicates that tendon length can be significantly increased when appropriate tension is applied to the tissues by the third week. Therefore, early passive motion should commence around the 10th day, followed by the introduction of early active joint motion in the subsequent phase, progressing up to the 21st day [30, 31].

In this period, to increase muscle strength, proximal stability, and distal mobility, closed kinetic chain exercises, capsule and muscle stretching exercises, dumbbell exercises against gravity, theraband, scapular stabilization exercises, and proprioceptive exercises are preferred (**Figures 3** and **4**). Physiotherapy applications such as

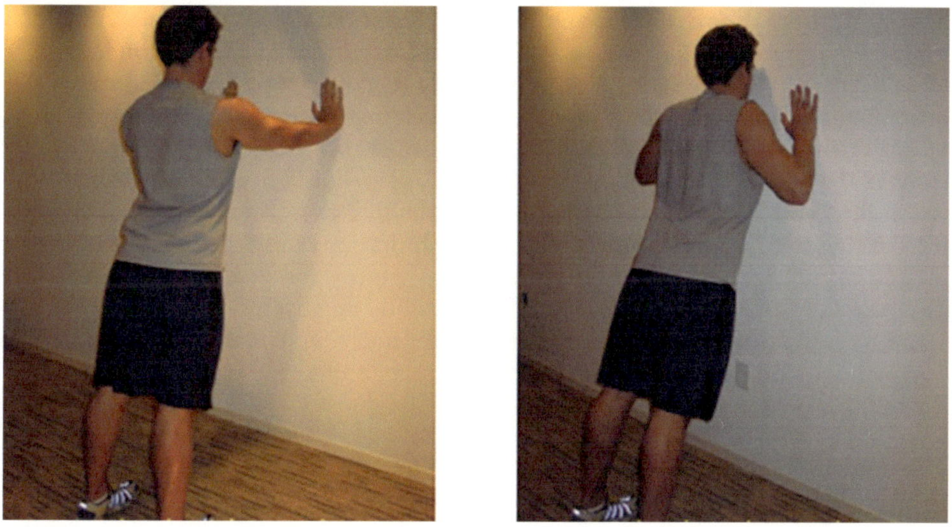

Figure 3.
Closed kinetic chain scapula retraction.

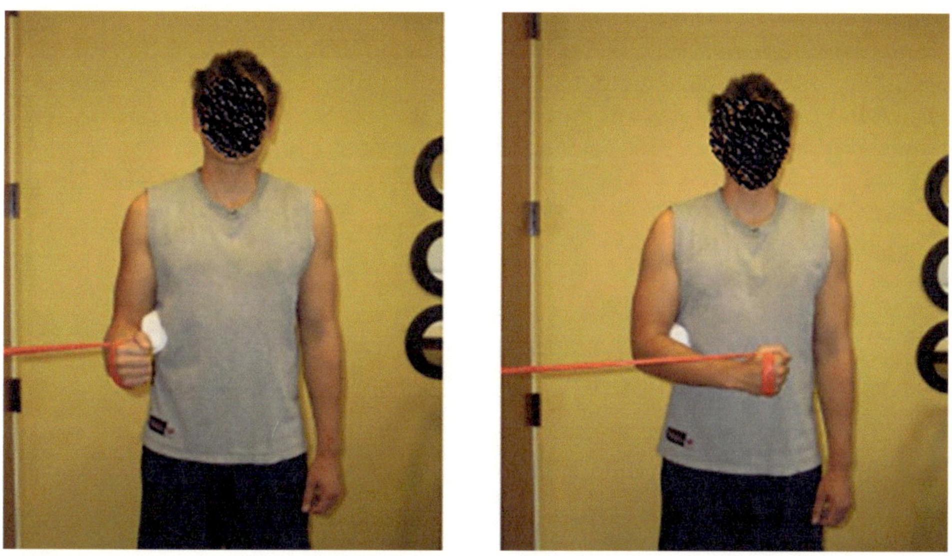

Figure 4.
Shoulder internal rotation strengthening.

ultrasound, electrical stimulation, hot applications, grade 3–4 humeral mobilization, and transverse friction massage can be used [32].

The aim of rehabilitation in this phase is to ensure the extension of newly synthesized collagen and to increase regular collagen formation. Collagen formation continues until the 6th week. Soft tissue mobilization performed on the tissue and its surroundings allows the incision scar to extend, proper muscle function and pain reduction [1, 24]. Restoration of scapular muscle activity is very important in this period for dynamic proximal stability [14].

During the chronic phase of advanced rehabilitation, the primary goals include achieving a full, painless, active range of motion, gradually restoring strength, power, and endurance in the glenohumeral and scapular regions, as well as facilitating a return to functional activities. Patients have experienced a reduction in pain and tenderness in the glenohumeral joint during rest; however, decreased scapular movement persists. By the sixth week, collagen formation starts to diminish gradually. Maturation or remodeling initiates in the third week and continues until approximately 12–18 months. Throughout this period, it is essential to maximize tissue extensibility, with a strong emphasis on strengthening exercises [33].

Returning to full activity without pain and limitations can take patients over a year, and regaining their full potential is often a lengthy and challenging process, both financially and emotionally. Therefore, establishing home exercise programs and maintaining patient follow-up are critical for individuals with RCT. Integrating a recommended home exercise program into most rehabilitation protocols is essential to ensure complete recovery.

6. Conclusions

The combination of physiotherapy with conventional treatment and exercise training for patients with rotator cuff tears (RCT) has been shown to yield positive outcomes in pain relief, functional activity, muscle architecture, and muscle strength. Given the nature of the lesions and muscle structure, integrating physiotherapy methods with exercise is crucial due to its clinical applicability, affordability, and accessibility, all of which contribute to effective improvements in shoulder muscle strength and tendon adaptation. Furthermore, these exercises are sustainable, as they can be easily incorporated and performed as home exercises.

Conflict of interest

The authors declare no conflict of interest.

Author details

Emine Merve Ersever
Ankara University Haymana Vocational School, Ankara, Turkey

*Address all correspondence to: merversever@gmail.com

References

[1] Kuhn JE. Exercise in the treatment of rotator cuff impingement: A systematic review and a synthesized evidence-based rehabilitation protocol. Journal Shoulder Elbow Surgery. 2009;**18**(1):138-160

[2] Lewis J. Rotator cuff related shoulder pain: Assessment, management and uncertainties. Manual Therapy. 2016;**23**:57-68

[3] Littlewood C. Contractile dysfunction of the shoulder (rotator cuff tendinopathy): An overview. The Journal of Manual & Manipulative Therapy. 2012;**20**:209-213

[4] Pope DP, Croft PR, Pritchard CM, Silman AJ. Prevalence of shoulder pain in the community: The influence of case definition. Annals of the Rheumatic Diseases. 1997;**56**:308-312

[5] Van der Windt DA, Koes BW, de Jong BA, Bouter LM. Shoulder disorders in general practice: Incidence, patient characteristics, and management. Annals of the Rheumatic Diseases. 1995;**54**:959-964

[6] Redondo-Alonso L, Chamorro-Moriana G, Jimenez-Rejano JJ, Lopez-Tarrida P, Ridao-Fernandez C. Relationship between chronic pathologies of the supraspinatus tendon and the long head of the biceps tendon: Systematic review. BMC Musculoskeletal Disorders. 2014;**15**:1-10

[7] Scott A, Squier K, Alfredson H, Bahr R, Cook JL, Coombes B, et al. ICON 2019: International scientific tendinopathy symposium consensus: Clinical terminology. British Journal of Sports Medicine. 2020;**54**:260-262

[8] Linaker CH, Walker-Bone K. Shoulder disorders and occupation. Best Practice & Research. Clinical Rheumatology. 2015;**19**:405-423

[9] Jancuska J, Matthews J, Miller T, Kluczynski MA, Bisson LJ. A systematic summary of systematic reviews on the topic of the rotator cuff. Journal of Orthopaedic & Sports Physical Therapy. 2018;**6**(9):23-25

[10] Miswan MF, Saman TS, Hui MZ, Al-Fayyadh MR. Correlation between anatomy of the scapula and the incidence of rotator cuff tear and glenohumeral osteoarthritis via radiological study. Journal of Orthopaedic Surgery (Hong Kong). 2017;**25**(1):230-949

[11] Sasiponganan C. Subacromial impingement anatomy and its association with rotator cuff pathology in women: Radiograph and MRI correlation, a retrospective evaluation. Skeletal Radiology. 2019;**48**(5):781-790

[12] Lewis JS. Rotator cuff tendinopathy: A model for the continuum of pathology and related management. British Journal of Sports Medicine. 2010;**44**:918-923

[13] Clark JM 2nd. Tendons, ligaments, and capsule of the rotator cuff. Gross and microscopic anatomy. JBJS. 1992;**74**(5):713-725

[14] Cook JL, Rio E, Purdam CR, Docking SI. Revisiting the continuum model of tendon pathology: What is its merit in clinical practice and research? British Journal of Sports Medicine. 2016;**50**:1187-1191

[15] Croisier JL, Foidart-Dessalle M, Tinant F, Crielaard JM, Forthomme B. An isokinetic eccentric programme for the management of chronic lateral

epicondylar tendinopathy. British Journal of Sports Medicine. 2007;**41**:269-275

[16] Wilson F, Walshe M, O'Dwyer T, Bennett K, Mockler D, Bleakley C. Exercise, orthoses and splinting for treating achilles tendinopathy: A systematic review with meta-analysis. British Journal of Sports Medicine. 2018;**52**:1564-1574

[17] Lim HY, Wong SH. Effects of isometric, eccentric, or heavy slow resistance exercises on pain and function in individuals with patellar tendinopathy: A systematic review. Physiotherapy Research International. 2018;**23**:e1721

[18] Almokhtar A, Mulla Z, Alqurashi A. Relationship between acromial anatomy and rotator cuff tears in Saudi Arabian population. Cureus. 2020;**12**(5):83-804

[19] Maruvada S, Madrazo-Ibarra A, Varacallo M. Anatomy, Rotator Cuff. Treasure Island (FL): Stat Pearls; 2021

[20] Vila-Dieguez O, Heindel MD, Awokuse D, Kulig K, Michener LA. Exercise for rotator cuff tendinopathy: Proposed mechanisms of recovery. Shoulder & Elbow. 2023;**15**(3):233-249

[21] Oliva F, Piccirilli E, Bossa M, Via AG, Colombo A, Chillemi C, et al. I.S.Mu.L.t - Rotator cuff tears guidelines. Muscles Ligaments and Tendons Journal. 2015;**5**:227-263

[22] Belletti M, Mallia L, Lucidi F, Reichmann S, Mastroianni C, De Marinis MG, et al. Complementary therapy and support services for formal and informal caregivers in italian palliative care hospices: An exploratory and descriptive study. Support Care Cancer. 2011;**19**:1939-1947

[23] Krischak G, Gebhard F, Reichel H, Friemert B, Schneider F, Fisser C, et al. A prospective randomized controlled trial comparing occupational therapy with home-based exercises in conservative treatment of rotator cuff tears. Journal of Shoulder and Elbow Surgery. 2013;**22**(9):1173-1179

[24] Vila-Dieguez O, Heindel MD, Awokuse D, Kulig K, Michener LA. Exercise for rotator cuff tendinopathy: Proposed mechanisms of recovery. Shoulder & Elbow. 2023;**15**(3):233-249

[25] Fu CJ, Sun JB, Bi ZG, Wang XM, Yang CL. Evaluation of platelet-rich plasma and fibrin matrix to assist in healing and repair of rotator cuff injuries: A systematic review and meta-analysis. Clinical Rehabilitation. 2017;**31**(2):158-172

[26] Fahy J, Lewis K. Large to massive rotator cuff tendon tears: A protocol for a systematic review investigating the effectiveness of exercise therapy on pain, disability and quality of life. Openal Research. 2021;**4**:65-69

[27] Desmeules F, Boudreault J, Dionne CE, Frémont P, Lowry V, MacDermid JC, et al. Efficacy of exercise therapy in workers with rotator cuff tendinopathy: A systematic review. Journal of Occupational Health. 2016;**58**(5):389-403

[28] Lewis JS. Rotator cuff tendinopathy. British Journal of Sports Medicine. 2009;**43**(4):236-241

[29] Littlewood C, Ashton J, Chance-Larsen K, May S, Sturrock B. Exercise for rotator cuff tendinopathy: A systematic review. Physiotherapy. 2012;**98**(2):101-109

[30] Boudreau N, Gaudreault N, Roy J-SS, Bédard S, Balg FFF, Bedard S, et al. The addition of glenohumeral adductor coactivation to a rotator cuff exercise

program for rotator cuff tendinopathy: A single-blind randomized controlled trial. Journal of Orthopaedic & Sports Physical Therapy. 2019;**49**:126

[31] Lin I, Wiles L, Waller R, et al. What does best practice care for musculoskeletal pain look like? Eleven consistent recommendations from high-quality clinical practice guidelines: Systematic review. British Journal of Sports Medicine. 2020;**54**:79-86. DOI: 10.1136/bjsports-2018-099878

[32] Salamh P, Lewis J. It is time to put special tests for rotator cuff–related shoulder pain out to pasture. Journal of Orthopaedic & Sports Physical Therapy. 2020;**50**(5):222-225

[33] Littlewood C, Malliaras P, Chance-Larsen K. Therapeutic exercise for rotator cuff tendinopathy: A systematic review of contextual factors and prescription parameters. International Journal of Rehabilitation Research. 2015;**38**(2):95-106

Section 4

Conservative Treatment Approaches

Chapter 6

Manual Therapy: A Cornerstone in the Treatment of Shoulder Injuries

Muhammad Hafeez, Shabana Rahim and Kiran Shahzadi

Abstract

Shoulder injuries, which can range from adhesive capsulitis to rotator cuff disorders, present substantial obstacles to physical therapy (PT) because of the complex anatomy and biomechanical requirements of the joint. One of the core interventions in physical therapy has long been acknowledged to be manual therapy (MT) when treating different shoulder injuries as a safe, non-surgical treatment approach. This chapter describes the role of different manual therapy techniques that can help patients with shoulder injuries regain their range of motion (ROM), manage pain, and improve movement functionality. The physiological consequences and clinical applications of several evidence-based manual procedures are highlighted, including soft tissue mobilizations (STM), joint mobilizations (JM), myofascial release (MFR), and muscle energy techniques (MET). It also emphasizes how crucial expert manual therapy techniques are to providing patient-centered care and maximizing recovery in shoulder rehabilitation, but it also poses some absolute and relative contraindications related to patient-specific conditions. The current chapter presents information about current challenges alongside future potential advancements together with its limitations in this field as an important guide for healthcare providers and patients pursuing total shoulder injury treatment.

Keywords: manual therapy, shoulder injuries, myofascial release, soft tissue mobilization, joint mobilization, muscle energy technique, pain management

1. Introduction

Humans possess one of the most adaptable and fragile shoulder joints in their body structure, which results in numerous regular injuries. Due to its delicate anatomy and extensive movement possibilities, the shoulder becomes at risk for developing rotator cuff tears along with impingement syndrome and adhesive capsulitis (AC) (also known as frozen shoulder) and dislocations. Proper management of shoulder conditions requires a full grasp of shoulder structures along with early and appropriate treatment of standard injuries.

1.1 Overview of common shoulder injuries

The shoulder joint ranks as one of the most frequent musculoskeletal conditions that affects people with differences in age and exercise ability. Movement functions of the shoulder joint depend on the four muscles within the rotator cuff as well as their corresponding tendons for joint stability. Rotator cuff tears (RCT) develop from endurance-based overhead activities as well as trauma and the aging-related degenerative changes [1]. Pain along with weakness combined with limitations in performing daily lifting or reaching activities form common symptoms of this issue.

Shoulder impingement syndrome (SIS) refers to a common condition that compresses rotator cuff tendons together with bursa bones under acromion structures during arm elevation motion. The condition develops because of problems with muscle balance or bad posture and repetitive movements [2]. Patients feel pain when they raise their arms, but if they do not receive treatment, their shoulder dysfunction can become long-term.

Adhesive capsulitis or frozen shoulder is a serious joint condition that features the development of stiffness and discomfort because of capsule swelling and inflammation. Medical experts have not determined the precise cause of this condition, yet doctors link it frequently to prolonged immobilization or diabetes or systemic health conditions [3]. A humeral head dislocation occurs due to forceful movement that separates it from the glenoid cavity leading to severe pain as well as instability problems alongside possible enduring complications including repeated dislocations and labral tears [4].

1.2 The complexity of shoulder anatomy and its susceptibility to injury

The shoulder bones have outstanding mobility capabilities due to their special structure, but achieve this through diminished joint stability. As the glenohumeral joint (GHJ) works as a ball-and-socket connection, its alignment and movement control depend heavily on soft tissue elements, including ligaments, tendons, and muscles for stability. The shoulder joint shows natural instability because its glenoid fossa is shallower than its large humeral head size [5].

Shoulder mechanical operations heavily depend on both the scapulothoracic joint function along with all surrounding shoulder musculature. Body movement abnormalities in the shoulder blade led to scapular dyskinesis (SD) that distorts shoulder complex stress distributions, thus making damage more likely [6]. The combination of unbalanced muscles with deficient neuromuscular control along with insufficient joint positioning ability makes shoulders more susceptible to sustaining harm.

1.3 Importance of early diagnosis and intervention

It is important to detect shoulder injuries early since it helps prevent permanent disability and leads to optimal healing outcomes. According to Brady, when medical care is delayed, patients may experience the development of secondary complications, which include muscle atrophy together with joint contractures and persistent pain syndromes [1]. A medical assessment must include histories, physical testing, and appropriate imaging exams to help healthcare professionals identify pathologies, which will help them select proper treatments.

Manual therapy plays a vibrant role in forming early intervention methods, which experts now consider fundamental. Manual therapy achieves dual functions because it treats symptom relief through soft tissue restriction management along with the treatment of underlying dysfunctional causes of the pathology [7]. Cellular joint motion combined with therapeutic exercises with patient education stands as the fundamental system of shoulder rehabilitation treatment.

2. Understanding manual therapy

The discipline of manual therapy uses therapist hand methods to examine diagnoses and heal musculoskeletal disorders (MSDs). The practice includes multiple treatment approaches that focus on stretching tissues while decreasing pain levels alongside the improvement of joint motion capacity and rehabilitation of proper body movements. The biomechanical and neurophysiological properties of the body form the foundation of manual therapy practice since they demonstrate how soft tissues link together with joints and the nervous system [8]. Shoulder injury treatment starts with manual therapy because this main treatment approach addresses deficits in both structure and function to achieve complete healing.

2.1 Definition and principles of manual therapy

According to the American Physical Therapy Association (APTA), skilled hand movements used during manual therapy provide physical treatment of joints and soft tissues to alter pain levels while improving ROM and reducing or eliminating inflammation from soft tissues and promoting relaxation and tissue repair while facilitating movement and enhancing functional abilities [9]. Manual therapy treatment operates on several fundamental principles that involve two main aspects.

Joint mobilization together with soft tissue manipulation functions to change mechanical tissue properties by breaking adhesion and stretching tight structures along with enhancing joint alignment.

Few primary therapeutic actions emerge from manual therapy since mechanoreceptors and nociceptors become stimulated, thus affecting pain perception while also resulting in hypertonic muscle relaxation [8].

Professional therapists apply manual therapy according to individual patient requirements through assessments of personal injuries while taking their functionality and therapeutic goals into account.

Manual therapy benefits complex shoulder areas due to its simultaneous treatment of various dysfunction aspects. Therapists can reach overall treatment targets when they merge these methods to provide their patients with pain minimization along with increased range of motion and better functional abilities.

2.2 Types of manual therapy techniques used for shoulder injuries

Medical practitioners use different manual treatment methods to treat shoulder injuries by focusing on various dysfunction types for rehabilitation purposes. The therapist applies various treatment methods, such as soft tissue mobilization, followed by joint mobilization and manipulation, alongside myofascial release accompanied by muscle energy techniques.

2.2.1 Soft tissue mobilization (STM)

The procedure of STM includes targeted movements and tension application upon muscles, tendons, ligaments, and fascia to eliminate tension while enhancing blood flow circulation and dissolving scar tissue. Shoulder muscle tightness combined with trigger points and myofascial restrictions can successfully treat these conditions using this particular therapy method [10]. The technique of soft tissue mobilization delivers benefits to wounded rotator cuff tendinitis patients by both increasing blood flow and decreasing inflammation, as well as easing tendon sensitivity. The rehabilitation therapist uses massage modalities like cross-friction massage and deep tissue massage to treat dysfunctional parts of the injured tissue.

2.2.2 Joint mobilization (JM) and manipulation

The process of JM uses calibrated forces on joints in order to normalize arthrokinematics motion patterns, which enhances joint range of motion. The different grades of these techniques determine their force amplitude along with their force velocity. Medical personnel use Grades I–II mobilizations to treat soreness as well as Grades III–IV mobilizations to promote joint flexibility and recover standard joint mechanics [11].

The performance of manipulation results in a high-velocity and low-amplitude force applied to a joint, which produces an audible cavitation sound. The practice of manipulation offers valuable treatment for patients with frozen shoulder conditions when it helps reduce capsular restrictions. The primary goal of both mobilization and manipulation techniques is to return glenohumeral joint mobility along with optimal scapulohumeral rhythm function according to the work of Giuseppe et al. [6].

2.2.3 Myofascial release (MFR)

A gentle sustained pressure application on fascial tissue through myofascial release enables tension release and allows for better tissue stretching. The presence of restricted fascial tissue often leads to abnormal shoulder motions that produce pain due to tissue injuries. MFR provides benefits to patients with adhesive capsulitis because it loosens joint capsules along with adjacent connective tissues, which promotes increased ROM and pain reduction [12]. The therapist implements this method in combination with additional manual therapy interventions for better results (**Figure 1**).

2.2.4 Muscle energy techniques (MET)

Therapists apply counterforces on patients to enhance mobility and increase muscle length through voluntary muscle contractions known as METs. The application of METs provides effective treatment for correcting shoulder muscle imbalances

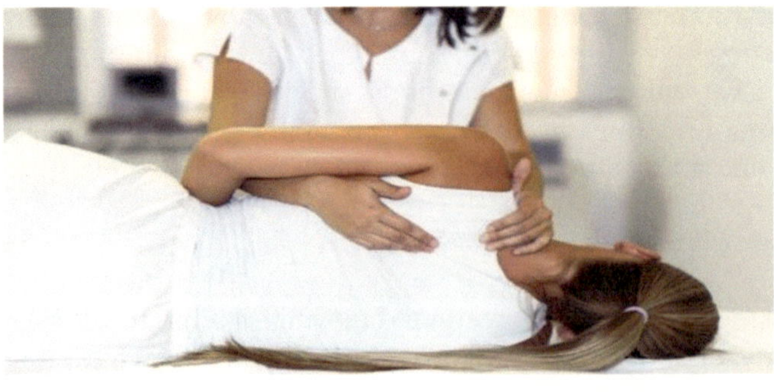

Figure 1.
Myofascial release therapy. (A young female patient is in side-lying position and receiving myofascial release therapy for her left shoulder) (https://massageblisschicago.com/myofascial-release-therapy-methodology-features/).

together with joint disorders. METs provide treatment in scapular dyskinesis by developing serratus anterior strength together with trapezius lower activation to counteract upper trapezius activation and levator scapulae activation [6]. This method enables better neuromuscular control as well as improved overall stability and shoulder complex coordination.

2.3 Role of manual therapy in pain relief, improving ROM, and restoring function

Shoulder injury rehabilitation includes extensive aspects of manual therapy, which minimize pain while improving ROM deficits and functional abilities through direct and indirect treatment effects.

The therapeutic actions of manual therapy both control pain signals through the neurophysiological mechanisms and activate the body's endogenous opioid response to minimize pain signals. When practicing soft tissue mobilization and joint mobilization, practitioners activate mechanoreceptors to both stop pain signals and create pain relief [7]. The reduction of inflammation and edema through manual therapy produces additional contribution to pain reduction.

Manual therapy works toward normal ROM recovery through treating joint hypomobility and soft tissue limitations and muscle tension. Direct application of joint mobilization and manipulation techniques enables patients to develop better arthrokinematics movements through simultaneous improvement of soft tissue compliance with myofascial release and manual soft tissue techniques. According to Fernandes [12], manual therapy significantly raises active and passive ROM in patients with frozen shoulder, thus allowing for meaningful shoulder function recovery.

Patients achieve functional restoration when manual therapy teams up with therapeutic exercises to teach neuromuscular skills. Manual therapy builds a structural base for muscle strengthening by improving joint function dimensions as well as muscle flexibility and neural control mechanisms. The addition of dynamic stabilization exercises enables patients to receive progressive treatment from scapular dyskinesis rehabilitation with METs and joint mobilization methods to better their shoulder stability and performance [6].

Manual therapy represents an adaptable, evidence-based solution for managing injuries that affect the shoulder. The therapeutic effects of manual therapy allow practitioners to deal with pain while managing restricted ROM and clinical function, thus becoming an essential rehabilitation resource. Other therapeutic approaches strengthen the application of manual therapy to provide complete patient outcomes for shoulder injury management.

3. Benefits of manual therapy for shoulder injuries

The various advantages of manual therapy help shoulder injury patients by treating both their symptoms and fundamental dysfunction causes of injury. The recreational benefits of manual therapy treatment include pain and inflammation relief while improving joint flexibility and mobility and strengthening muscles as well as enhancing coordination. Furthermore, the speedy recovery of patients enables them to return to their daily routines or sports activities. As part of a whole rehabilitation process, manual therapy works to speed up healing and produce better functional results, thus allowing patients to recover their independence and maintain their quality of life (QOL).

3.1 Reduction of pain and inflammation

Manual therapy immediately benefits patients through its successful reduction of pain and inflammation, which frequently appear as symptoms of shoulder injuries. All three manual therapy techniques of soft tissue mobilization with joint mobilization and myofascial release focus on treating nociceptive pathways alongside inflammatory processes that produce discomfort. The practice of soft tissue mobilization cuts down localized inflammation through enhanced lymphatic drainage and boosted circulation, which eliminates swelling and edema [10]. The application of low-grade oscillations during joint mobilization activates mechanoreceptors in the joint capsule that control the transmission of pain signals through the gate control theory (GCT) of pain modulation [8].

Neurophysiological changes activate immediate pain relief, which lets patients become more involved with therapeutic exercises. The therapy helps decrease muscle guarding and hypertonicity because these factors commonly increase pain while restricting joint motion. The healing process and recovery become more efficient when manual therapy treats multiple factors affecting the healing environment. Fernandes described manual therapy treatments as successfully decreasing pain intensity for patients suffering from rotator cuff tendinitis and adhesive capsulitis and post-surgical shoulder conditions [12].

The pain relief achieved through manual therapy makes patients more comfortable and helps them follow rehabilitation instructions, which leads to improved long-term recovery results. Improvement in joint mobility and flexibility for shoulder injuries create joint hypomobility, which restricts the ROM because of capsular tightness and adhesions between joints along with muscle imbalances. The direct structural limitations get resolved through manual therapy, which restores joint range of motion along with flexibility. The Grades III and IV joint mobilization techniques demonstrate high effectiveness for improving shoulder accessory movements that support typical shoulder mechanics [11]. The combination of joint mobilization with stretching exercises successfully increases both active and passive ROM in patients with frozen shoulder because it enables normal shoulder function (**Figure 2**) [3].

Soft tissue mobilization together with myofascial release helps treat the restricted musculature and fascial tissue to enhance flexibility even more. Such techniques reduce fibrotic tissue while improving tissue elasticity to reduce stiffness, which

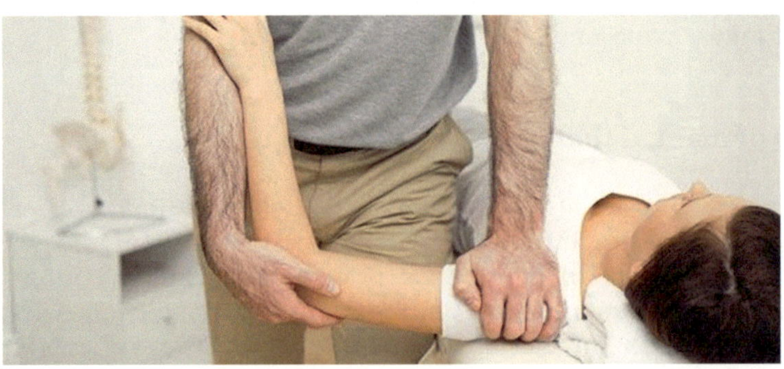

Figure 2.
Shoulder joint manipulation. (A female patient suffering from left frozen shoulder is lying supine and being treated by a physical therapist in order to improve shoulder ROM) (https://ultimatehealthclinic.ca/blog/osteopathy-tips-and-news/can-osteopathy-help-treat-frozen-shoulder/).

allows users to achieve better movement coordination. The extensive range of motion that results from improved joint mobility along with better flexibility diminishes both medical symptoms while minimizing the chances of developing secondary injuries, including altered movement routines. The recovery of proper joint function through manual therapy delivers both therapeutic and permanent advantages for joint health.

3.2 Enhancement of muscular strength and coordination

The common aftermath of shoulder injuries includes muscle weakness and poor neuromuscular control, which develops because of pain inhibition or disuse or through altered movement patterns.

Manual therapy, when performed with therapeutic exercises, functions effectively to boost the strength of muscles and improve neuromuscular coordination patterns in patients. The activation of weak muscles combined with antagonist inhibition through METs stands out as an effective method [6]. Physical therapy professionals use METs to activate the serratus anterior and lower trapezius muscles in patients with shoulder dysfunction since these muscles are usually underactive in scapular dyskinesis cases. These techniques boost the patient's scapular stability and alignment, which consequently leads to superior overall shoulder function and less occurrences of repeated injuries. Manual therapy helps patients develop better proprioceptive abilities because this ability is essential for executing complex shoulder movements. Manual therapy methods that include joint mobilization together with soft tissue mobilization activate mechanoreceptors, which improve both sensory information transmission and motor control abilities [7].

The dual benefits of better muscle activation along with enhanced body positioning lead patients toward smooth movements that protect vulnerable tissues over the long term. Through its dual approach to strength development and coordination training, the treatment ensures patients recover their physical abilities and acquire injury prevention abilities. Promotion of Faster Recovery and Return to Daily Activities or Sports Manual therapy achieves its most important aim through quickened healing processes which enable patients to go back safely into their sport or daily routines.

The treatment combination of pain reduction with joint mobility recovery and muscle strength improvement establishes healing conditions during rehabilitation period. Active players and athletes gain special benefit from fast recovery since long periods of rest can make them lose their conditioning and decrease their sports performance.

Studies demonstrate that rehab programs that include manual therapy end up reducing the duration of shoulder injury recovery periods. The combination of exercise therapy with manual therapy helped rotator cuff tendinitis patients reach pre-injury activity levels more quickly compared to patients who received exercise therapy only, according to the work of Brady et al. [1]. Shoulder rehabilitation outcomes after surgery demonstrate enhancement when manual therapy treatments are implemented because patients achieve faster recovery of ROM and strength development [4].

Manual therapy creates an approach to recovery that enables patients to actively participate in their rehabilitation process. Additional home-based exercises unite with clinical treatments to offer continuous care that leads patients to maintain their rehabilitative advancement. By putting patients at the center of treatment, the recovery time decreases alongside better compliance to rehabilitation guidelines, which produces superior results.

4. Assessment before manual therapy

A complete clinical examination must precede manual therapy applications to shoulder injuries in order to conduct safe and effective medical interventions. A complete diagnosis requires both historical data collection and physical tests, as well as diagnostic imaging examinations. It is essential to identify all contraindications for manual therapy since this assessment will help prevent worsening of injuries alongside adverse effects. The assessment procedure serves to select correct rehabilitation techniques and creates initial measurement points which enable monitoring of treatment progress.

4.1 Importance of a thorough clinical evaluation

Clinical evaluations that provide a complete examination form the basis for creating specific treatment approaches that suit each patient's requirements. The therapist uses this method to identify the root cause of the condition while assessing how severe the damage is and what elements contribute to the problem, including imbalances between muscles and joint dysfunction or postural issues [13].

Manual therapy becomes ineffective or potentially dangerous when this evaluation step is omitted. The evaluation process starts with gathering complete patient information about symptom characteristics and their timing along with known causes and treatment history. The diagnosis and treatment expectations improve when medical professionals understand if the pain developed suddenly or evolved gradually as well as if it resulted from an accident or emerged without explanation.

The evaluation process includes activity-related inquiries about work and daily functions to detect functional limits, which guide rehabilitation targets. Evaluation of patient psychosocial characteristics, which include movement anxiety (kinesiophobia) and injury-associated nervousness, stands equally important to the assessment process. The recovery process and treatment adherence are both heavily affected by various factors [1].

The therapist delivers complete healthcare by understanding and treating both physical and mental health needs of patients. Diagnostic Tools and Tests for Shoulder Injuries: A physical examination follows the historical assessment to provide doctors with diagnostic and treatment decision-making information through objective findings. A shoulder complex evaluation consists of observational components and palpation along with motion range tests and strength measures and tests that assess particular shoulder structures.

4.1.1 Observation

During both static and dynamic movements, the therapist will examine the patient for proper posture and alignment of their scapula and the symmetry of their shoulders. Examples of shoulder injury indications include forward head posture or winged scapulae or asymmetrical shoulder levels, which show potential biomechanical contributions to the injury [6].

4.1.2 Palpation

By using palpation, the therapist can detect both swollen and tight muscles along with sensitive tissue areas. A doctor can use tenderness tests to evaluate rotator cuff involvement by assessing the greater tuberosity, while anterior joint line tenderness points to labral pathology [5].

4.1.3 Range of motion testing

The assessment includes both active and passive range of motion measurements that check joint movement along with tracking any movement limitations. Passive ROM testing by therapists differentiates from active ROM testing by patients to determine mechanical from neuromuscular dysfunction causes. The assessment of active ROM compared to passive ROM determines whether muscle weakness or inhibition exists, while joint hypomobility or capsular tightness becomes apparent from passive ROM restrictions [11].

4.1.4 Strength testing

Manual muscle testing (MMT) serves to assess the strength of shoulder muscles, which include deltoid and rotator cuff as well as scapular stabilizers. According to Giuseppe, the weakness of particular shoulder muscles including supraspinatus and serratus anterior helps identify treatment areas [6].

4.1.5 Special tests

Specialized tests exist for identifying particular conditions affecting the shoulder. Examples include: The assessments of Neer's Test and Hawkins-Kennedy Test help determine the presence of subacromial impingement syndrome. The supraspinatus tendon integrity can be evaluated using the Empty Can Test (Jobe's Test). The evaluation includes Speed's Test, which checks for biceps tendinitis with Yergason's Test used to detect labral tears.

- Apprehension test: Identifies instability or risk of dislocation. Imaging studies play an essential part alongside physical examination because they help doctors confirm their diagnoses and eliminate severe health conditions.

- Common imaging modalities include: X-rays, which help doctors identify fractures as well as dislocations and osteoarthritis while showing symptoms of calcific tendinitis. MRI produces detailed images of tendons along with ligaments and the labrum, which enables healthcare providers to detect rotator cuff tears and labral injuries and adhesive capsulitis [3].

Real-time examination of active structures through ultrasound (US) enables clinicians to see the rotator cuff and biceps tendon during procedures such as injections and aspiration. Magnetic resonance arthrography (MRA) should be used as an advanced imaging technique to evaluate complex intra-articular pathologies in patients [4].

5. Identifying contraindications for manual therapy

The safety and effectiveness of manual therapy exist until opposite indications appear, which demand specific modifications to maintain patient safety. The assessment process requires a thorough examination of contraindications for proper patient care. Absolute and relative contraindications exist for manual therapy according to their severity and risks to patient safety.

- *Absolute contraindications:* Manual therapy poses serious risks to patients in these particular conditions, thus becoming completely prohibited for use. Examples include:

    - o Acute fractures or dislocations.

    - o Active infections or inflammatory conditions, such as septic arthritis or rheumatoid arthritis flare-ups.

A severe case of osteoporosis elevates the possibility of developing pathological fractures. The treatment of unstable spinal cord injuries or neurological deficits should be avoided because manipulation procedures may intensify their condition.

- *Relative contraindications:* Manual therapy can be appropriate for these medical situations, although practitioners need to exercise careful judgment while modifying their techniques. Examples include:

The application of manual therapy should be avoided when patients have undergone recent surgical procedures or suffered traumatic injuries, since excessive force might harm healing tissues. The excessive joint mobility of these patients makes them vulnerable to joint subluxations and unstable joint positions. The treatments could be harmful to patients who suffer from vascular conditions, consisting of deep vein thrombosis (DVT) or arterial insufficiency, because pressure or movement could affect their circulation. The healing process and treatment response of patients with systemic diseases including diabetes and cancer may be negatively affected. Physical therapists must adjust their treatment methods for patients who present relative contraindications to lower the risks involved. The use of gentle mobilization techniques combined with soft tissue approaches replaces high-paced manual methods, and treatment should wait for the resolution of acute healing periods [7].

6. Manual therapy works best when used in conjunction with additional treatment methods as part of their rehabilitation approach

The maximum benefits of manual therapy appear when rehabilitation programs include complete approaches that recognize diverse aspects of shoulder injuries. Clinicians should use manual therapy in conjunction with exercise therapy and physical modalities as well as psychological support for a complete recovery method. The section analyzes how these supporting therapeutic approaches boost the success of manual therapy by achieving the best functional recovery result and sustaining patient health throughout life.

6.1 Integration with exercise therapy and rehabilitation programs

The basic principle of shoulder rehabilitation relies on exercise therapy that strengthens its association with manual therapy to treat muscular imbalances and establish stable joints while improving functional movements. The benefits from manual therapy treatment grow stronger through exercise therapy, which adds muscle strengthening along with neuromuscular control and dynamic stability training.

6.1.1 *Synergistic effects*

Manual therapy develops a beneficial circumstance for exercise because it reduces pain symptoms while boosting range of motion abilities. Muscle and joint mobilization techniques along with soft tissue procedures decrease pain while making exercise practice more comfortable for patients [1].

Exercise therapy boosts manual therapy effects through its ability to treat weak muscles and fix scapular dyskinesis. Patients reduce the risk of instability and lose gains in mobility by performing rotator cuff and deltoid and scapular stabilizer strengthening exercises to meet functional requirements.

6.1.2 *Examples of combined interventions*

6.1.2.1 *Rotator cuff tendinitis*

Cross-friction massage (CFM) and joint mobilization manual therapy techniques both minimize tendon inflammation and achieve better glenohumeral joint mechanics.

Therapy with elastic bands or weights helps patients recover strength and endurance in the supraspinatus, infraspinatus, and teres minor muscles.

6.1.2.2 *Adhesive capsulitis*

Joint mobilizations together with myofascial release techniques help release capsular restrictions, which leads to enhanced ROM improvements.

To keep improvements from physical therapy ongoing, patients should combine stretching exercises like wall climbing with towel stretches together with deltoid and rotator cuff muscle strengthening exercises.

6.1.3 *Clinical considerations*

Exercise therapy needs to progress alongside how the patient recovers from their condition. The recovery process consists of simple ROM exercises for early-phase therapy, which transitions to advanced dynamic stability and strengthening exercises [6]. The patient benefits from systematic integration of exercise therapy with manual therapy methods to reach the maximum outcomes.

Medical practitioners apply ultrasound treatment with heat and cold modalities and electrical stimulation techniques next to standard manual therapy interventions.

Manual therapy receives additional benefit through physical modalities, which help healing processes and minimize pain and enhance patient comfort. The applied modalities produce secondary physiological benefits, which support the mechanical and neurophysiological approaches of manual therapy.

6.1.4 *Ultrasound therapy*

The tissue-healing process benefits from ultrasound technology that creates high-frequency sound waves to improve blood circulation and reduce inflammation together with collagen stimulation.

Medical staff can administer ultrasound treatment to rotator cuff tendinitis or bursitis patients before doing manual therapy to enable better tissue responsivity for mobilization and manipulation. Scientists demonstrated that ultrasound treatment with manual therapy enhances tendon healing and speeds up patient recovery, according to Jacob [3].

6.1.5 Heat and cold therapy

The application of heat enhances tissue elastic capabilities and creates relaxation, which makes it the best option as a pre-treatment tool for manual therapy interventions. People who apply warm packs to stiff shoulder muscles before joint mobilizations achieve better treatment results because these packs make the tissues easier to manipulate.

The application of ice packs serves two purposes following aggressive manual therapy techniques or exercise work to both reduce inflammation and block acute pain signals.

6.1.6 Electrical stimulation

Transcutaneous electrical nerve stimulation (TENS) employs low-voltage electrical currents which both alter pain transmission pathways and activate substance P release from the body. TENS therapy teaming up with manual therapy techniques produces quick pain reduction that enables patients to better accept hand-driven techniques.

The application of Interferential Current Therapy (IFC) on deep tissues proves effective for diminishing inflammation and supporting shoulder healing in individuals with adhesive capsulitis or post-surgical shoulder stiffness.

6.1.7 Clinical considerations

Modalities operate to boost manual therapy outcomes, yet they should not act instead of active rehabilitation measures, especially exercise therapy. Modalities serve their best purpose when they help manual therapy reach its maximum effectiveness and create better clinical results for patients [7].

7. Psychological support and patient education for holistic recovery

Shoulder injuries result in important psychological effects together with social impacts through frustration, while patients experience anxiety and fear about potential new injuries. People need psychological support in combination with education about their health condition to obtain complete recovery from their issues.

7.1 Psychological support

The development of both fear avoidance behaviors and kinesiophobia leads patients with chronic shoulder pain to reduce their involvement in rehabilitation activities. Grade exposure to movements combined with positive reinforcement using Cognitive-behavioral techniques provides effective solutions to address such barriers.

DOI: http://dx.doi.org/10.5772/intechopen.1011018

A rehabilitation program achieves better success when patients receive emotional backing together with achievable targets, as this creates both motivation and adherence. The therapist's consistent feedback together with their encouragement maintains the patient's dedication to recovery.

7.2 Patient education

The rehabilitation process becomes more effective when patients receive instruction about their injury's anatomy, combined with pathology and healing process information, since this creates active patient involvement. Understanding the pain-alleviating effects and mobility benefits of manual therapy builds trust between patient and therapist leading to better patient-therapist cooperation.

The education of self-care, stretching, and strengthening exercises, which patients learn outside the clinic, helps maintain their continued recovery. By teaching patients how to position their bodies and construct proper workstations and exercising caution with their activities, patients will minimize the chances of re-injuring themselves.

7.3 Holistic benefits

A therapeutic approach that integrates manual therapy with psychological support along with patient education allows the treatment of physical and emotional aspects of recovery. Using this integrated approach, patients achieve better short-term results, yet it strengthens their ability to handle future medical challenges and health conditions [13].

8. Challenges and limitations of manual therapy

The high effectiveness of shoulder injury management through manual therapy techniques has important challenges together with specific limitations. Patients should understand the potential hazards and unfavorable reactions alongside the exclusion criteria and the mandatory expertise of qualified therapists along with their ongoing professional learning. It is necessary to comprehend these elements to achieve secure treatments with successful results.

8.1 Potential risks and complications if not performed correctly

Erroneous application of manual therapy creates specific risks, which intensify previously existing medical problems or produce fresh injuries to the patient. Furthermore, proper execution of hands-on procedures demands both accurate delivery of force and sufficient knowledge of tissue safety limits. Not following these principles may cause various adverse consequences among patients.

8.1.1 Tissue damage

Laboratory tests reveal that aggressive tissue mobilization pressure produces inflammations while muscle tears and tissue bruises can potentially occur. Aggressive cross-friction massage application to inflamed tendons causes increased irritation because it delays healing, according to Schleip [10].

High-velocity joint maneuvers, when executed improperly, can produce ligament sprains together with labral tears and increase joint instability, primarily among people who have hypermobility and pre-existing joint looseness.

8.1.2 Nerve injury

Joint mobilization techniques become unsafe when practitioners use improper joint positions or apply excessive pressure because this might squeeze or irritate surrounding nerves. Posterior-to-anterior glenohumeral joint moves with unstabilized position can compress the axillary nerve, causing temporary weaknesses and numbness of the deltoid muscle [11].

8.1.3 Increased pain and inflammation

Excessive manual physical therapy approaches generate inflammatory reactions that make patients experience enhanced pain sensations and swelling together with stiffness. Such methods create additional problems for patients experiencing acute injuries and those recovering from surgery because their tissues already show signs of damage.

8.1.4 Patient discomfort and anxiety

Lack of effective communication with patients along with failure to gain their consent may trigger concerns about discomfort or uncertainty and distrust. High-velocity manipulations might trigger patients' psychological distress about the treatment method because they can be considered aggressive by patients, which reduces their commitment to continuing therapy.

8.2 Mitigation strategies

A safe outcome demands that therapists complete patient evaluations before developing customized treatments, which require continuous assessment of patient reactions. The protocol uses incremental mobilization techniques together with gentle manipulation procedures during acute stages to provide safety measures until treatment intervention progression happens [7].

There are specific clinical scenarios where manual therapy treatment proves inappropriate.

Professional manual healthcare treatments must avoid use or need extensive change as part of particular clinical circumstances. Public health professionals must decode these circumstances before proceeding with patient treatment to prevent either injury or breaches of professional ethics.

8.2.1 Fractures and acute injuries

Manual therapy poses contraindications for performing therapy on patients who suffer from acute fractures along with dislocations or those presenting severe ligamentous injuries, since the healing tissues could become compromised by manipulation or mobilization treatment techniques. Medical research indicates that applying manual mobilization techniques on a fractured humerus will delay bone union and potentially produce improper alignment [4].

8.2.2 Severe osteoporosis

Treatment of patients with severe osteoporosis raises their chances of suffering pathological fractures because their bones have weakened. The delivery of normal or below-normal joint force during manual techniques can generate structural pathologies like compression fractures when treating patients with skeletal conditions.

8.2.3 Active infections or inflammatory conditions

The practice of manual therapy needs to be prohibited when a patient shows signs of active infections, which include septic arthritis (SA) or rheumatoid arthritis (RA) flares. The practice of touching inflamed or infected joints poses a risk that both infection spread and exacerbated inflammation could harm the joints [12].

8.2.4 Vascular and neurological conditions

Medical professionals should exercise full caution when treating patients with vascular insufficiency or deep vein thrombosis (DVT) along with peripheral neuropathy. Moving or applying pressure to areas in the vicinity of affected areas may harm circulation systems or intensify neurological problems.

8.2.5 Hypermobility and instability

People who experience joint hypermobility along with shoulder instability face intensified symptoms when receiving aggressive stretching or joint manipulation treatment. Solid joint performance and stability should be pursued by directing patients toward therapeutic exercise treatments [6].

8.3 Relative contraindications

The therapy remains an option when adapted to specific situations. Medical staff can apply gentle mobilization techniques to patients who have mild osteoarthritis (OA) or post-surgical stiffness through ranges without pain while obtaining prior patient authorization [11].

Proficient manual therapy deliverers along with ongoing professional expertise development represent key factors in this field.

A practitioner needs advanced knowledge and skills along with expert-level ability to successfully perform manual therapy. Manual therapy exists as both a clinical skill and scientific art, which demands complete mastery of understanding human anatomy combined with proficiency in hand-based therapeutic methods.

8.3.1 Technical proficiency

Overcoming manual therapy techniques requires training of great duration and dedicated practice. The practitioner needs to practice feeling tissue alterations alongside applying force with accuracy and making treatment modifications according to patient feedback. The ability to differentiate between capsular restrictions and muscular tightness needs advanced palpation expertise and logical clinical strategies [13].

8.3.2 Clinical decision-making (CDM)

There are several prerequisites to efficient manual therapy, which include properly analyzing assessments with established treatment ambitions to decide the right interventions. Professionals need critical thinking skills combined with problem-solving competencies to treat patients who have both rotator cuff tendinitis and scapular dyskinesis.

8.3.3 Continuous professional development

Continuous progress in manual therapy exists because researchers discover new techniques and publish fresh research findings at a steady rate. To remain in practice, practitioners need to dedicate themselves to ongoing learning activities which help them keep knowledge about evidence-based treatment approaches. Professional competence relies on three key elements, which include attendance at workshops and completion of advanced certifications like Orthopedic Manual Physical Therapy together with participation in peer discussions as described in Grieve's Modern Musculoskeletal Physiotherapy [7].

8.3.4 Ethical responsibility

Healthcare practitioners should recognize what they cannot treat optimally so they can properly refer patients to specialist teams. Therapists who suspect a labral tear or complex adhesive capsulitis must work with orthopedic surgeons or sports medicine physicians to deliver full care to patients.

8.4 Impact on patient outcomes

Patients achieve better results from practitioners who dedicate themselves to constant knowledge improvement and follow modern evidence-based guidance instead of depending only on unscientific beliefs. After receiving training in advanced manual therapy, therapists demonstrate better patient outcomes by achieving greater satisfaction while patients heal more quickly [1].

9. Future directions in manual therapy for shoulder injuries

The discipline of manual therapy adjusts because of emerging technological discoveries and research findings alongside a growing priority of evidence-based practice. The modern developments in practice guide medical practitioners to handle shoulder injuries in ways that deliver superior treatment quality while amplifying patient participation throughout the recovery process. The evaluation discusses contemporary trends in manual therapy methods and technological developments of VR and robotics platforms, further using evidence-based practice to develop advanced treatment methods.

9.1 Emerging trends and innovations in manual therapy techniques

Manual therapy now experiences a transition toward specialized methods that utilize contemporary biomechanical insulation besides neurophysiological and tissue scientific advancements. The innovations attempt to enhance treatment accuracy together with variation reduction to produce optimal patient results.

9.1.1 Targeted soft tissue interventions

Real-time soft tissue structure observation through ultrasound and elastography tools gives therapists opportunities to check patient tissue structures. Medical professionals can identify tendon tears and fascial restrictions correctly through this method to apply targeted, specific rehabilitation techniques [10].

9.1.2 Neuromodulatory techniques

Research on manual therapy neurophysiology allowed scientists to produce neuromodulatory approaches and proprioception enhancement methods. Neurodynamic mobilizations represent a novel therapeutic approach that focuses on advancing nerve mobility while lowering neural tension, especially when treating conditions with radicular symptoms or nerve entrapment [8].

9.1.3 Hybrid techniques

Healthcare providers now adopt success by using traditional manual procedures along with additional treatment techniques, including dry needling, along with instrument-assisted soft tissue mobilization (IASTM). The utilization of combined methods in treatment takes advantage of various intervention benefits to treat intricate symptoms. The combination of joint mobilizations with IASTM techniques leads to faster patient recovery when treating individuals with adhesive capsulitis, according to research by Fernandes [12].

9.1.4 Patient-Centered customization

Manual therapy has adopted personalized medicine methods to create treatment approaches that respect individual patient features such as physical abilities and health conditions along with age groups. Treatment methods under this approach provide long-term sustainability in addition to their established effectiveness.

9.2 Widespread research evaluates technology integration in manual therapy practice

Modern manual therapy has experienced a revolutionary advancement through technological integration because this development delivers improved accuracy together with patient-specific adaptive practices that extend across large patient groups. New technologies including virtual reality systems together with robotic devices and wearable technology are examined because of their ability to boost rehabilitation success and recovery.

9.2.1 Virtual reality (VR)

The virtual reality technology creates virtual environments, which duplicate actual physical activities to make rehabilitation exercises more interesting and compelling for patients. The virtual reality system takes patients through shoulder range of motion exercises by providing real-time feedback about their exercise execution [14]. The therapy enables distant monitoring by therapists as well as improves patient adherence while simultaneously supporting tele-rehabilitation standards.

9.2.2 Robotics-assisted therapy (RAT)

The use of robotic devices continues to increase for helping with joint mobilizations and strengthening of muscles during physical therapy. The devices provide accurate force control and speed management and directional control, which lead to precise interventions with identical results throughout. The RAT approach demonstrates success in glenohumeral joint mechanics improvement for frozen shoulder patients as demonstrated through findings comparable to manual therapy techniques [15]. Mathematical technology demonstrates useful applications in post-surgical recovery processes by enabling precise delivery of healing-inducing stress requirements.

9.2.3 Wearable sensors and biofeedback

Maximum movement patterns and ROM together with muscle activation data become measurable through sensors which integrate accelerometers and gyroscopes in wearable devices. The obtained data allows therapists to improve their manual therapy methods while helping monitor patient advancements through time. Patients receive warnings from biofeedback systems that trigger when their scapular stabilization exercises deviate from proper movement guidelines, thereby improving neuromuscular control, according to the work of Brady et al. [1].

9.2.4 Telehealth platforms

Telehealth programs now extend manual therapy support to people located in underserved locations and remote settings. Patients can conduct self-mobilization exercises with guidance from therapists through video consultations combined with digital tools in spite of the limited replication of hands-on techniques remotely. The combined healthcare approach brings both ongoing patient care support and technology-driven overcoming of distance limitations.

9.3 Importance of evidence-based practice in advancing treatment protocols

Evidence-based practice (EBP) functions as the fundamental principle that advances manual therapy since its interventions must derive from scientifically proven and clinically applicable sources. EBP keeps its essential position in healthcare development by validating new techniques while optimizing current treatment procedures with the goal of solving existing problems in medical understanding.

9.3.1 Systematic reviews and meta-analyses

Systematic reviews combined with meta-analyses supply thorough evaluations about how manual therapy works in treating rotator cuff tendinitis alongside adhesive capsulitis and other particular conditions. Research studies enable practitioners to determine effective care methods while showing exactly where extra evaluation is needed [1]. Recent meta-analyses reinforce manual therapy treatment together with exercise therapy by validating its position as an established clinical practice.

9.3.2 Randomized controlled trials (RCTs)

Randomized controlled trials serve as the primary method to determine new treatment effectiveness as well as their level of superiority against existing procedures. Ongoing research involving robotic shoulder rehabilitation protocols against traditional manual therapy in post-surgical care delivers positive preliminary findings [15].

9.3.3 Clinical guidelines and protocols

APTA together with other professional bodies produces continuous updates of clinical guidelines through evidence-based analysis. Use of these guidelines helps practitioners follow current best practices because they provide standards for treatment protocols [9].

9.3.4 Interdisciplinary collaboration

Clinical advancement of manual therapy demands integrated efforts between medical personnel including practitioners and researchers together with technicians and engineers. Multiple fields collaborating gives the discipline the capacity to combine different proficiencies which enables the creation of new solutions for unmet requirements. According to Banyai, physical therapists who work with biomedical engineers created state-of-the-art robotic devices for joint mobilizations [15].

9.3.5 Patient-Centered outcomes research

Research initiatives should direct their focus toward assessing outcomes which matter to patients through measures such as quality of life together with functional independence and return to their desired activities including work and sports. Elaborating the full impact manual therapy possesses on patients' lives will provide validation that interventions have both effective results and meaningful meaning.

10. Conclusions

The management of shoulder injuries depends strongly on manual therapy, which serves as an adaptable, evidence-based approach to handle pain and improve both functional results and restore mobility. Manual therapy techniques, which include soft tissue mobilization, provide extensive benefits because they address multiple impairments of shoulder pathologies while giving quick pain relief that extends beyond short-term treatment. The fundamental value of manual therapy appears in its ability to connect naturally with exercise protocols and physical medicine approaches and psychological elements for designing complete rehabilitation plans.

When patients accept manual therapy within their entire treatment approach, their healing process speeds up and their quality of life enhances, alongside a reduced susceptibility to re-injury. Therapeutic excellence requires therapists to both acquire hands-on capabilities and monitor modern treatment trends, which leads to the provision of advanced clinical standards. Manual therapy presents multiple difficulties because it requires experts and precise contraindication evaluation as well as constant professional education. Evidence-based practice and interdisciplinary approaches prove essential in establishing new treatment standards because of these identified factors.

Managed development in rehabilitation requires ongoing research together with training to reach the complete potential of manual therapy practices. Advanced treatment approaches can emerge through studies about technology applications and enhanced manual therapy methods and neurophysiological mechanisms in order to create more effective medical care methods. Establishing a setting that embraces original thinking will maintain manual therapy as an essential part of musculoskeletal healthcare, thus enabling patients and practitioners to reach their most effective results.

Manual therapy stands as a vital therapeutic method to treat shoulder injuries because it connects established medical practices with innovative healthcare developments. Shoulder dysfunction treatment requires sustained collaborative support for education and research investment to help people with shoulder dysfunction problems. Through collective efforts, we will redefine rehabilitation boundaries to restore hope, function, and resilience in people all across the world.

Acknowledgements

The author would like to sincerely thank respected colleagues for their constant encouragement, critical feedback, and intellectual support throughout the development of this chapter on *"Manual Therapy: A Cornerstone in the Treatment of Shoulder Injuries."* Their mutual knowledge and attitude of cooperation significantly improved the quality of this academic work.

Additionally, special thanks are also extended to junior faculty members, whose passion, diligence, and helpful criticism were crucial in refining the content and guaranteeing its applicability to both academic and clinical practice.

The author also appreciates the broader professional community for creating an atmosphere that supported ongoing education and knowledge sharing, which provided the groundwork for this scholarly effort.

Conflict of interest

The authors declare no conflict of interest.

Author details

Muhammad Hafeez*, Shabana Rahim and Kiran Shahzadi
Department of Physical Therapy Agile Institute of Rehabilitation Sciences, Bahawalpur, Pakistan

*Address all correspondence to: drhafeezarain@gmail.com

References

[1] Brady N, Dejaco B, Lewis J, McCreesh K, McVeigh JG. Physiotherapist beliefs and perspectives on virtual reality supported rehabilitation for the management of musculoskeletal shoulder pain: A focus group study. PLoS One. 2023;**18**(4):e0284445. DOI: 10.1177/20552076241234738

[2] Platt BN, Sullivan BM, Dripchak S, Uhl TL, Sciascia AD, Kibler W, et al. A plague of their own: Injury incidence remains elevated in the 2021 Major League Baseball season compared to pre-COVID-19 seasons. International Journal of Sports Physical Therapy. 2022;**17**(6):1104. DOI: 10.26603/001c.38479

[3] Jacob L, Gyasi RM, Koyanagi A, Haro JM, Smith L, Kostev K. Prevalence of and risk factors for adhesive capsulitis of the shoulder in older adults from Germany. Journal of Clinical Medicine. 2023;**12**(2):669. DOI: 10.3390/jcm12020669

[4] Kavaja L, Lähdeoja T, Malmivaara A, Paavola M. Treatment after traumatic shoulder dislocation: A systematic review with a network meta-analysis. British Journal of Sports Medicine. 2018;**52**(23):1498-1506. DOI: 10.1136/bjsports-2017-098539

[5] Neumann DA. Neumann's Kinesiology of the Musculoskeletal System-E-Book. St. Louis, Missouri: Elsevier Health Sciences; 2024. Available from: https://www.google.com.pk/intl/en/about/products?tab=ph

[6] Giuseppe LU, Laura RA, Berton A, Candela V, Massaroni C, Carnevale A, et al. Scapular dyskinesis: From basic science to ultimate treatment. International Journal of Environmental Research and Public Health. 2020;**17**(8):2974. DOI: 10.3390/ijerph17082974

[7] Selfe J, Greenhalgh S, Mercer C, Finucane L. Red Flags. Grieve's Modern Musculoskeletal Physiotherapy E-Book; 2024. p. 248

[8] Bialosky JE, Bishop MD, Price DD, Robinson ME, George SZ. The mechanisms of manual therapy in the treatment of musculoskeletal pain: A comprehensive model. Manual Therapy. 2009;**14**(5):531-538. DOI: 10.1016/j.math.2008.09.001

[9] American Physical Therapy Association. Guide to Physical Therapist Practice 4.0; 2023. Available from: https://www.apta.org

[10] Schleip R. Fascial plasticity–a new neurobiological explanation part 2. Journal of Bodywork and Movement Therapies. 2003;**7**(2):104-116. DOI: 10.1016/S1360-8592(02)00076-1

[11] Hengeveld E, Banks K. Maitland's Vertebral Manipulation: Management of Neuromusculoskeletal Disorders-Volume 1. London, UK: Elsevier Health Sciences; 2013

[12] Fernandes MR. Adhesive capsulitis: Current concepts. Musculoskeletal Surgery. 2025:1-10. DOI: 10.1007/s12306-025-00897-7

[13] Sueki DG, Cleland JA, Wainner RS. A regional interdependence model of musculoskeletal dysfunction: Research, mechanisms, and clinical implications. The Journal of Manual & Manipulative Therapy. 2013;**21**(2):90-102. DOI: 10.1179/2042618612Y.0000000027

[14] Clark WE, Sivan M, O'Connor RJ. Evaluating the use of robotic and virtual reality rehabilitation technologies to improve function in stroke survivors: A narrative review. Journal of Rehabilitation and Assistive Technologies Engineering. 2019;**6**:2055668319863557. DOI: 10.1177/2055668319863557

[15] Banyai AD, Brișan C. Robotics in physical rehabilitation: Systematic review. Healthcare (MDPI.). 29 Aug 2024;**12**(17):1720. DOI: 10.3390/healthcare12171720

Section 5

Advanced Surgical Interventions

Chapter 7

Superior Capsular Reconstruction Using Autologous Long Head of the Biceps Tendon: A Cost-Effective and Biomechanically Reliable Option for Managing Massive Rotator Cuff Tears

Kyun-Ho Shin, Seung-Beom Han and Il-Tae Jang

Abstract

Large-to-massive rotator cuff tears (LMRCTs) represent one of the most challenging conditions in shoulder surgery, with conventional arthroscopic repair techniques demonstrating consistently high failure rates. Superior capsular reconstruction (SCR) has emerged as a promising joint-preserving technique for LMRCTs, but traditional grafts—such as fascia lata autografts and dermal allografts—are associated with increased costs and donor site morbidity. The long head of the biceps tendon (LHBT) has recently gained attention as an autologous graft option for SCR. It is readily available within the operative field, eliminating the need for additional incisions, graft preparation, or allograft use. This chapter examines SCR using the autologous LHBT (LHBT-SCR) as an alternative approach for managing irreparable LMRCTs and reviews biomechanical studies, surgical technique, and clinical outcomes. Biomechanical studies demonstrate that LHBT-SCR provides greater resistance to humeral head migration and restores superior shoulder stability. Early clinical evidence supports its effectiveness, with improved range of motion, reduced retear rates, and high patient satisfaction. When used as a pedicled graft with preserved glenoid attachment, the LHBT maintains its native vascularity, potentially enhancing graft viability and healing. This technique is compatible with standard arthroscopic portals and instruments. Proper patient selection is essential, with emphasis on biceps tendon quality and subscapularis integrity. LHBT-SCR offers a cost-effective, biologically sound alternative to conventional SCR.

Keywords: arthroscopy, rotator cuff injuries, joint-preserving surgery, superior capsular reconstruction, biceps brachii

1. Introduction

Large-to-massive rotator cuff tears (LMRCTs) are among the most challenging conditions encountered in shoulder surgery [1–5]. These tears, often involving multiple tendons and characterized by tendon retraction, muscle atrophy, and fatty infiltration, present substantial obstacles to traditional repair techniques [1, 2, 4, 6, 7]. The underlying pathophysiology includes both mechanical disruption at the tendon-bone interface and progressive biological degeneration, including altered joint kinematics and muscular atrophy [4, 8, 9].

Retrospective studies have consistently reported high failure rates following arthroscopic repair of LMRCTs. Galatz et al. observed a 94% retear rate at 2 years following complete arthroscopic repair of massive tears, while Boileau et al. reported that only 71% of supraspinatus repairs achieved tendon healing [6, 7]. Despite advances in arthroscopic technique, reported structural failure rates continue to range from 30% to 94%, largely dependent on tear chronicity, tissue quality, and patient-related factors [1, 2].

In relatively younger or physiologically active patients with preserved glenohumeral joint space and functional range of motion, joint preservation becomes the preferred strategy [3, 5, 10]. These patients often do not yet meet criteria for arthroplasty but suffer from pain and loss of function due to irreparable defects [3, 5, 10].

While reverse total shoulder arthroplasty (RTSA) is an accepted salvage procedure in elderly patients, its application in younger individuals is limited by its complication profile, finite implant longevity, and irreversible alteration of native biomechanics [3, 5, 10–14]. RTSA also precludes future biological reconstruction, making it a less favorable option in patients who wish to preserve native shoulder anatomy [3, 5, 10–14].

Given these limitations, the development of joint-preserving biological reconstruction techniques has gained increasing attention. These include partial repair, tendon transfers, and patch augmentation. Among these, superior capsular reconstruction (SCR) has emerged as a promising strategy to restore superior stability and preserve shoulder kinematics in patients with irreparable posterosuperior rotator cuff tears (RCTs) [15, 16]. However, conventional SCR techniques often involve the use of autologous fascia lata or dermal allografts, which are associated with increased cost, donor site morbidity, or variable graft integration [17–23].

More recently, the autologous long head of the biceps tendon (LHBT) has been proposed as an alternative graft source for SCR. Easily accessible during standard shoulder arthroscopy, LHBT eliminates the need for separate graft harvest or costly allograft materials, and biomechanical studies have demonstrated its ability to restore superior glenohumeral stability [24–26].

This chapter aims to provide a comprehensive overview of SCR using the autologous LHBT, referred to hereafter as LHBT-SCR. It will examine the biomechanical rationale, surgical technique, patient selection criteria, clinical outcomes, and remaining challenges associated with this technique, and position it as a viable joint-preserving option for managing irreparable LMRCTs.

2. Joint-preserving surgical options

Several joint-preserving surgical options exist for managing irreparable LMRCTs, each with distinct advantages and limitations depending on the specific tear pattern, patient characteristics, and surgeon preference.

Partial repair focuses on restoring the anterior-posterior force couple by repairing the intact portions of the rotator cuff, even when a complete repair is not possible. This technique, pioneered by Burkhart and colleagues, aims to improve joint mechanics and function rather than achieve complete anatomical restoration [1, 2]. The partial repair typically involves margin convergence techniques, where the edges of the tear are brought together to reduce tension at the repair site [1, 2]. While this approach can improve pain and function in approximately 65–80% of cases, long-term outcomes may be limited by progressive tear extension and continued superior migration of the humeral head [1, 2, 27–29].

Tendon transfer procedures offer another joint-preserving solution, particularly for irreparable posterosuperior tears, by redirecting functional muscle-tendon units to substitute for deficient rotator cuff components. The latissimus dorsi transfer, one of the most widely used techniques, reroutes the latissimus tendon to compensate for the lost function of the infraspinatus and teres minor, especially in younger patients experiencing external rotation weakness [30–32]. The pectoralis major transfer is generally indicated for anterosuperior tears associated with subscapularis insufficiency [33, 34]. More recently, the lower trapezius transfer has been utilized to address posterosuperior defects and has shown encouraging results in restoring external rotation [35]. Despite their functional benefits, tendon transfers involve technically demanding procedures, require prolonged rehabilitation, and may be associated with donor site morbidity. Furthermore, surgical success is highly dependent on appropriate patient selection and meticulous technique [3, 5, 10].

Patch augmentation and spacer devices represent additional joint-preserving options, particularly useful for bridging large defects or reinforcing partial repairs. Dermal allografts provide a biologic scaffold for tissue ingrowth while offering immediate mechanical support [36, 37]. Xenografts, commonly derived from porcine or bovine tissues, serve a similar purpose but have raised concerns due to higher retear rates and potential immunologic reactions [38]. Synthetic patches, composed of durable polymeric materials, are engineered to offer long-term mechanical stability but may provoke inflammatory responses in some cases [39]. As an alternative, subacromial balloon spacers have been introduced as a minimally invasive method for reducing superior humeral head migration and decreasing subacromial friction. In a recent study, Gomes et al. also reported promising short-term outcomes for subacromial resurfacing using fascia lata autograft as another solution for irreparable tears [40]. However, the long-term durability, cost-effectiveness, and biological compatibility of both patches and spacers remain subjects of ongoing debate and investigation.

2.1 SCR

SCR has emerged as a promising technique for irreparable LMRCTs. This procedure reconstructs the superior capsule of the glenohumeral joint using a graft (autograft or allograft) attached medially to the superior glenoid and laterally to the greater tuberosity. This reconstructed structure helps prevent superior migration of the humeral head and restores shoulder biomechanics [15, 16]. The detailed technique and specific evidence will be discussed extensively in subsequent sections.

2.2 Summary of joint-preserving options

See **Table 1**.

Technique	Advantages	Disadvantages	Ideal candidates
Partial repair	• Technically familiar • Preserves remaining tissue • Less invasive	• High retear rate • Limited long-term outcomes • May not prevent superior migration	• Partially reparable tears • Preserved anterior-posterior balance • Minimal superior migration
Tendon transfer	• Addresses muscle deficiency • Can restore active function • Potential durable results	• Technical complexity • Donor site morbidity • Extended rehabilitation	• Young, active patients • Specific functional deficits • Good quality recipient tissue
Patch augmentation	• Reinforces weak tissue • Provides scaffold for healing • Addresses gap in tissue	• Cost • Variable integration • Potential inflammatory response	• Younger patients • Cuff tendon deficiency • Good bone quality
Balloon spacer	• Minimally invasive • Quick recovery • Reversible	• Temporary solution • Limited long-term data • May deflate/dislocate	• Elderly patients • Temporary pain relief needed • Poor candidates for larger procedures
SCR (allograft)	• Biomechanically favorable • Preserves future options • Addresses superior instability	• Cost • Technical demands • Variable tissue integration	• Irreparable superior tears • Minimal arthritis • Good remaining cuff function

Table 1.
Joint-preserving surgical options for the management of large-to-massive rotator cuff tears.

3. SCR: Concept and evidence

3.1 Historical development

The concept of SCR was first introduced by Teruhisa Mihata and colleagues in the early 2010s [15, 16]. In a series of biomechanical cadaveric studies published in 2012, Mihata et al. demonstrated that reconstruction of the superior capsule could effectively restore superior stability in shoulders with irreparable LMRCTs [15]. This groundbreaking work redefined the functional anatomy of the shoulder by emphasizing the superior capsule's crucial role in limiting superior translation of the humeral head—a stabilizing function that had previously been attributed almost exclusively to the rotator cuff tendons [15].

In a subsequent clinical study published in 2013, Mihata and colleagues reported promising early outcomes using autologous fascia lata grafts for SCR [16]. Their surgical technique involved harvesting a thick fascia lata graft, typically 6 to 8 mm in thickness, and securing it from the superior glenoid to the greater tuberosity. This construct functioned as a static restraint against the superior migration of the humeral head. Clinically, patients demonstrated marked improvements in forward elevation (from 84° to 148°) and external rotation (from 26° to 40°), along with substantial gains in American Shoulder and Elbow Surgeons (ASES) scores (from 23.5 to 92.9), indicating both symptomatic relief and functional restoration.

3.2 Biomechanical rationale

The biomechanical principles underpinning SCR are multifactorial [15, 41, 42]. First, the reconstructed capsule serves as a static restraint against superior humeral head migration, re-establishing central joint stability and restoring glenohumeral alignment [15, 41, 42]. Second, by restoring this central stability, SCR facilitates the preservation of the anterior-posterior force couple—specifically, the coordinated function of the subscapularis anteriorly and the infraspinatus and teres minor posteriorly. This restored balance allows for more effective muscle activation during shoulder movement [15, 41, 42]. Third, the procedure enhances deltoid efficiency. This central stabilization restores the deltoid's mechanical advantage by optimizing its length-tension relationship, thereby improving its mechanical advantage in generating arm elevation [15, 41, 42]. While SCR functions as a passive stabilizer, it does not constrain dynamic shoulder motion. Glenohumeral mechanics remain physiologic, supporting coordinated arm elevation and rotation. Multiple cadaveric studies confirm that a properly executed SCR closely replicates the kinematics of an intact shoulder, supporting its biomechanical validity [15, 41, 42].

3.3 Graft options

Multiple graft materials have been investigated for use in SCR, each offering distinct biomechanical and biological profiles. Fascia lata autografts, originally described by Mihata, are typically 6 to 8 mm in thickness and provide excellent tensile strength and biological incorporation. However, they necessitate an additional harvest site, potentially increasing operative time and donor site morbidity [15, 17]. Human dermal allografts, such as ArthroFlex, offer substantial thickness (usually 2 to 4 mm) and eliminate the need for autograft harvest. These grafts are convenient and reduce surgical trauma, but they are associated with higher costs, and questions remain regarding their long-term integration and remodeling [18–23]. More recently, the LHBT has emerged as a promising alternative. Readily available within the surgical field, the LHBT can be used without additional incisions or graft preparation, offering advantages in terms of cost-effectiveness and surgical efficiency [24–26, 43]. Finally, synthetic grafts have also been explored as an alternative option in SCR. These materials are associated with a risk of foreign-body reactions and exhibit inconsistent rates of biological integration. To enhance both mechanical strength and biological incorporation, synthetic patches are often combined with fascia lata autografts in a layered or hybrid configuration [44, 45].

3.4 Clinical outcomes of SCR using fascia lata or dermal allografts

SCR using fascia lata or dermal allografts has shown generally favorable outcomes in irreparable posterosuperior RCTs, though results are influenced by graft type, surgical technique, and patient factors. Mihata et al. reported dramatic improvements with fascia lata autografts, including increases in ASES scores from 23.5 to 92.9 and forward elevation from 84° to 148°. MRI confirmed intact grafts in 83% of patients, correlating with better outcomes [16]. In a comparative study, Takayama and Ito found that elderly patients treated with Teflon grafts achieved forward elevation of 151°, comparable to 164° in the TFL group, with nearly identical pain scores (NRS 1.0 vs. 0.9) and acromiohumeral distances (8.3 vs. 7.5 mm) [23]. Lacheta et al. evaluated dermal allograft SCR in 22 patients and reported improvement in ASES scores from 54.0 to 83.9, along with a reduction in VAS pain scores from 4 to 0 [21]. Radiographically, the acromiohumeral distance increased from 7.0 to 8.3 mm, and graft integrity on MRI exceeded 75% across evaluated sites. Interestingly, clinical outcomes did not show a strong correlation with graft integrity status [21]. Burkhart et al. followed 41 patients for 34 months, reporting ASES score gains from 52 to 90 and sustained improvements in external rotation (+11°). Graft healing was seen in 85%, though 19% failed to reach the minimal clinically important difference in ASES score, and 5% required revision [20, 22]. In contrast, Woodmass et al. reported limited benefit in a high-risk cohort, with 22 early failures among 34 patients. Failure was particularly common in revision cases, patients with subscapularis tears, high infraspinatus fatty infiltration, female sex, and those treated by low-volume surgeons [19]. Pennington et al. reported significant improvements in range of motion and strength in 86 patients treated with dermal allograft SCR [18]. ASES scores increased from 52 to 82, forward flexion improved from 120° to 160°, and abduction from 103° to 159°. Radiographic evaluation showed an increase in the acromiohumeral interval from 7.1 to 9.7 mm, and 90% of patients reported overall satisfaction with the outcome [18]. In summary, SCR provides reliable structural and functional improvement in selected patients, with fascia lata offering the most consistent results. Dermal allografts remain a widely used alternative but demonstrate greater variability, particularly in complex or revision cases.

4. Rationale for using the LHBT in SCR

4.1 Rationale

The LHBT offers several compelling advantages as a graft choice for use in SCR, distinguishing it from both other autografts and allografts [24–26, 43]. Its appeal lies in surgical efficiency—repurposing tissue already present in the operative field to address multiple pathologies simultaneously [24–26, 43].

First, using the LHBT as an autograft eliminates the need for separate donor site harvest [24–26, 43]. Unlike fascia lata grafts requiring a thigh incision, with added pain and scarring, the LHBT can be accessed directly through the same standard shoulder portal used during arthroscopic evaluation [24–26, 43]. For the operating surgeon, this intraoperative accessibility eliminates the need for graft preparation outside the operative field, significantly reducing surgical time and technical complexity [24–26, 43].

Economically, LHBT autografts are significantly more cost-effective than commercial dermal allografts. In a matched cohort study of 132 patients, the use of a dermal patch increased total surgical costs by $4930 ($P < .001$), even after adjusting for surgical and clinical variables [46]. These added expenses are often not fully reimbursed by insurers. In contrast, the LHBT involves no additional material cost, making it particularly attractive in resource-limited healthcare systems [46].

The technique is especially valuable in patients with biceps pathology, which is found in 80–92% of LMRCTs [47]. Rather than performing a separate biceps tenodesis or tenotomy for symptomatic biceps pathology, the LHBT-SCR technique simultaneously addresses both the rotator cuff deficiency and the biceps lesion—effectively transforming what would otherwise be discarded as a "waste product" into a structurally valuable reconstruction graft [24–26, 43].

As autologous tissue, the LHBT avoids risks of inflammatory reaction, infection, and disease transmission associated with allografts. It is already biologically adapted to the patient, which may support more reliable graft healing [24–26, 43]. Additionally, when the LHBT is left attached at the glenoid origin, it functions as a pedicled graft with preserved vascular supply [24–26, 43]. This vascularity may enhance biologic incorporation and long-term viability compared to avascular grafts [24–26, 43].

4.2 Biomechanical evidence

Biomechanical research has offered important insights into the structural and functional characteristics of the LHBT autografts in comparison to other graft materials commonly used in SCR, particularly regarding load-bearing capacity, stability, and the ability to restore native shoulder biomechanics [24, 48].

In a cadaveric study under static loading conditions, El-Shaar et al. evaluated the performance of the LHBT-SCR against reconstructions using tensor fascia lata (TFL) grafts in specimens with superior capsule deficiency [24]. The LHBT construct required approximately 393% of the force needed to produce superior humeral head translation compared to the deficient state, whereas the TFL graft required about 194%, indicating markedly greater resistance to superior migration. While this finding highlights the potential of the LHBT as a superior stabilizer, the use of static cadaveric testing limits its direct clinical applicability.

Supporting these results, Han et al. examined an SCR technique that preserved the LHBT in situ, maintaining its native glenoid attachment while securing the distal tendon to the greater tuberosity [48]. By retaining the tendon's vascular and neural elements, their cadaveric model demonstrated reduced subacromial contact pressures and re-established glenohumeral stability, while preserving physiologic joint motion [48]. However, these biomechanical results were derived from non-cyclic loading scenarios and may not fully replicate the demands of a physiologically active shoulder.

While these cadaveric biomechanical studies highlight the potential of the LHBT graft, their translation into clinical durability remains contingent upon patient-specific biological and mechanical factors [24, 48]. Further investigation in dynamic, physiologically loaded models and longer-term clinical follow-up studies is necessary to confirm their real-world effectiveness. A potential limitation of this method lies in the relatively limited width and surface area of the LHBT, which may be insufficient for covering extensive capsular defects. Nevertheless, technical adaptations such as tendon spreading or reinforcement using residual rotator cuff tissue have been proposed to mitigate this constraint [24–26, 48].

4.3 Clinical evidence specific to the LHBT-SCR

While conventional SCR techniques have a more established clinical track record, the application of the LHBT as a graft in SCR is a relatively recent approach with emerging evidence supporting its efficacy. The studies summarized below focus specifically on the LHBT-SCR, highlighting its unique clinical outcomes apart from those seen with other graft materials. Chiang et al. reported a graft failure rate of 5.6% at 1 year postoperatively following LHBT-SCR. Notably, even in cases of graft failure, patients demonstrated acceptable clinical outcomes without major symptomatic complaints [49]. Rhee et al. emphasized the importance of the LHBT quality and tear extent in predicting outcomes [25]. When the LHBT with partial tearing involving more than 50% of the tendon was used, the postoperative retear rate of the rotator cuff reached 35.7%, underscoring the need for careful intraoperative evaluation of graft integrity [25].

Barth et al. conducted a comparative analysis involving 82 patients with massive posterosuperior RCTs who underwent one of three procedures: SCR using the LHBT (n = 24), double-row repair (n = 28), or transosseous-equivalent repair with patch augmentation (n = 30) [50]. At 24 months, patients with healed grafts in the LHBT-SCR group showed superior improvements in shoulder strength and also scored higher on clinical outcome scales, including Constant, ASES, SST, SSV, and VAS, compared to those with structural failure [50].

Llinás et al. evaluated 106 patients with a minimum of 2 years of follow-up, comparing conventional arthroscopic repair (AR; n = 50) to LHBT-SCR (n = 56) [51]. The LHBT-SCR group demonstrated a significantly lower retear rate (14.3%) compared to the AR group (46%) [51]. Additionally, the LHBT-SCR group had better clinical outcomes, with higher ASES scores (77.2 ± 7.5 vs. 71.0 ± 9.3), lower VAS pain scores (1.64 ± 1.03 vs. 2.12 ± 1.06), and improved active forward elevation (155° vs. 150°) and abduction (150° vs. 120°) [51].

Additionally, Kawashima et al. followed 22 patients for at least 2 years, comparing outcomes between LHBT-SCR (n = 12) and arthroscopic partial repair (APR; n = 10) [52]. Although the LHBT group showed greater improvement in forward flexion (160° vs. 134°), ASES (89.3 vs. 83.4), and UCLA scores (32.5 vs. 29.8), these differences did not reach statistical significance [52]. However, the acromiohumeral interval was significantly greater in the LHBT group (7.5 vs. 5.8 mm), indicating improved superior joint stability [52]. Retear rates were also lower in the LHBT group (42%) compared to the APR group (80%) [52]. Furthermore, a higher proportion of patients in the LHBT group achieved clinically meaningful improvements, including minimal clinically important difference (MCID), substantial clinical benefit, and patient-acceptable symptomatic state [52]. Specifically, 83% of patients reached the MCID for ASES scores, and all patients achieved MCID in UCLA scores [52].

A recent meta-analysis by Shin et al. systematically reviewed outcomes from six comparative studies involving 456 patients with LMRCTs, of whom 210 underwent LHBT-SCR and 246 received conventional RCR [43]. The pooled results demonstrated that LHBT-SCR significantly reduced the retear rate (OR = 0.21) and yielded greater improvements in forward flexion (SMD 0.32) and acromiohumeral interval (SMD 0.61), compared to conventional repair techniques [43]. Although no significant differences were observed in postoperative ASES, Constant, or UCLA scores, the authors concluded that LHBT-SCR offers a safe and effective option for LMRCTs, with added benefits in tendon integrity and superior joint stability [43].

While most studies report favorable outcomes with LHBT-SCR, the variability in study design—including retrospective vs. prospective methodology, sample size, follow-up duration, and definition of graft integrity—limits direct comparability. Moreover, subgroup differences based on surgical technique (e.g., single- vs. double-row repair), tendon quality (e.g., intact vs. degenerative LHBT), and fixation methods may significantly influence outcomes. Therefore, these encouraging early results should be interpreted with caution. The clinical efficacy of LHBT-SCR remains promising but must be tested across broader populations and surgical settings. Future prospective trials should prioritize stratifying outcomes by tendon integrity, tear configuration, and subscapularis status, all of which appear to influence graft behavior.

DOI: http://dx.doi.org/10.5772/intechopen.1011091

5. Surgical technique: Step-by-step approach to LHBT-SCR

LHBT-SCR combines elements of standard arthroscopic rotator cuff repair techniques with specialized steps for biceps harvest and utilization. The following describes a systematic approach to the procedure.

5.1 Patient selection

5.1.1 Primary indications

The fundamental prerequisite for considering LHBT-SCR is the presence of an irreparable LMRCT. Irreparability is typically defined by:

- Tendon retraction to the glenoid level (Patte grade 3)
- Significant muscle atrophy (Goutallier grade 3–4 fatty infiltration)
- Static superior migration of the humeral head
- Failed previous repair attempts

The procedure is particularly well-suited for younger and middle-aged patients (typically under 70 years) who wish to maintain native joint anatomy and preserve future treatment options. Critically, LHBT-SCR requires the presence of a viable LHBT with good tissue quality.

5.1.2 Contraindications

Several conditions represent relative or absolute contraindications to LHBT-SCR:

5.1.2.1 Absolute contraindications

- Complete absence or rupture of the LHBT
- Severe degenerative changes to the LHBT (marked thinning or calcification)
- Advanced glenohumeral arthritis (Hamada stage 3 or higher)
- Significant superior glenoid bone loss
- Irreparable subscapularis tears (completely destabilized force couples)

5.1.2.2 Relative contraindications

- Advanced age (>75 years) with low functional demands
- Pseudoparalysis with passive elevation <90°
- Significant medical comorbidities limiting rehabilitation potential

- Low rehabilitation compliance
- Severe osteoporosis limiting anchor fixation potential

5.2 Surgical procedure

An overview of the key surgical steps is illustrated in **Figure 1**, which summarizes the technical workflow of LHBT-SCR, from arthroscopic evaluation to tendon fixation and rotator cuff reinforcement.

5.2.1 Patient positioning and portal setup

The procedure is carried out with the patient in either the lateral decubitus or beach chair position, depending on surgeon preference and patient characteristics. Arthroscopic access is achieved using standard portals for rotator cuff repair: Standard posterior portal, Posterolateral viewing portal, Anterior portal through the rotator interval, and Lateral working portal for tuberosity preparation and anchor placement. No additional or specialized portals are required for this technique, making it readily adaptable for surgeons familiar with standard arthroscopic shoulder procedures.

5.2.2 Intra-articular evaluation and LHBT assessment

A thorough diagnostic arthroscopy must be performed at the outset. This critical step involves evaluation of all intra-articular pathology, including synovitis, labral lesions, and chondral damage. The subscapularis tendon must be carefully inspected, as any repairable tears should be addressed either intra-articularly or in the subacromial space before proceeding with the reconstruction. Special attention to LHBT is critical, as its integrity determines the feasibility of the entire procedure. Tendons with less than 50% partial tearing may still be suitable, whereas more extensive tearing or anchor, particularly in the setting of non-Type II SLAP pathology, warrants the use of alternative graft materials. This comprehensive evaluation allows the surgeon to make a final determination regarding proceeding with LHBT-SCR versus alternative procedures. These assessments, in conjunction with preoperative imaging, help determine whether to proceed with LHBT-SCR or opt for a different reconstructive approach.

5.2.3 Mobilization of the LHBT

Once the tendon is deemed suitable, it is mobilized by releasing the transverse humeral ligament along the bicipital groove and debriding the tendon back to healthy tissue, removing any frayed or degenerated segments. It is essential to confirm that it glides freely over the greater tuberosity, ensuring sufficient mobility for subsequent rerouting and fixation (**Figure 1A**).

5.2.4 Preparation of a neo-groove

A defining technical step in this procedure involves selecting an optimal site on the lateral aspect of the greater tuberosity and creating a shallow "neo-groove" using a burr. This groove serves as the seating channel for the rerouted LHBT. Care must

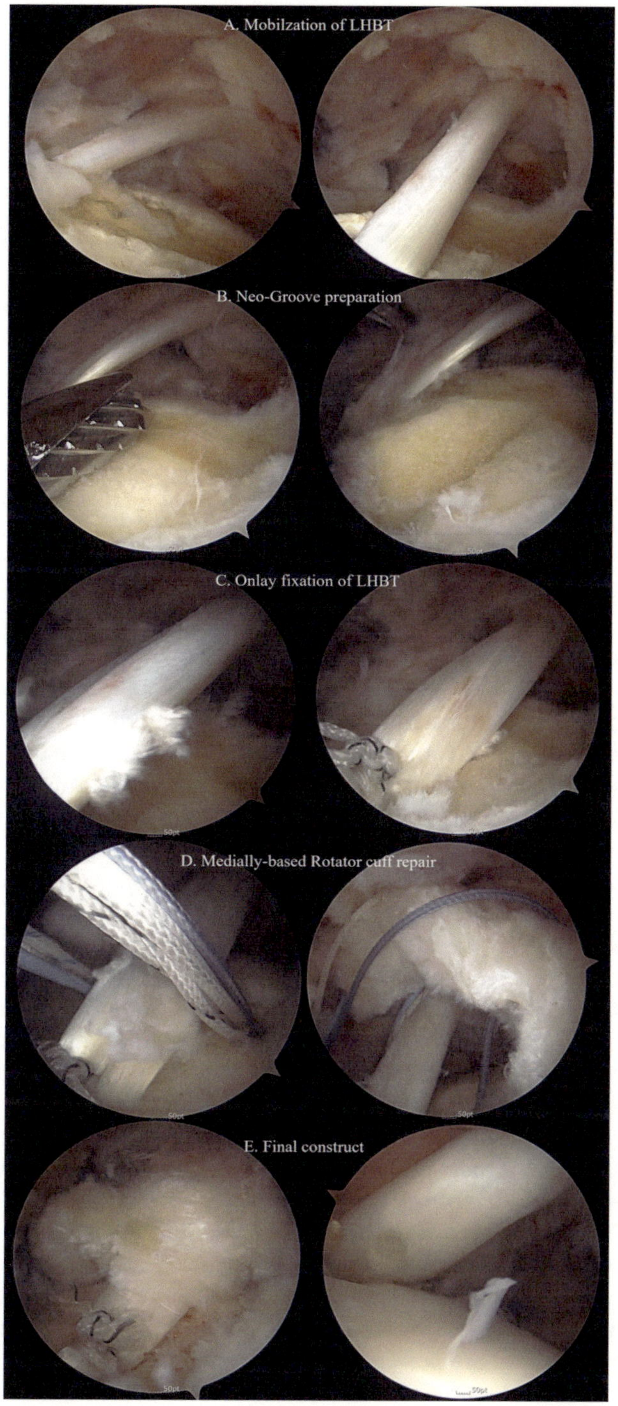

Figure 1.
Stepwise schematic of arthroscopic LHBT-SCR. This diagram illustrates the sequential technical steps in LHBT-SCR: (A) mobilization of the LHBT by releasing the transverse humeral ligament along the bicipital groove; (B) preparation of a neo-groove on the greater tuberosity; (C) anchor-based onlay fixation of the LHBT with appropriate tensioning; (D) medially based rotator cuff reinforcement over the graft; and (E) final construct shown from both subacromial and intra-articular views. Abbreviation: LHBT, long head of the biceps tendon; LHBT-SCR, superior capsular reconstruction using the autologous long head of the biceps tendon.

be taken not to over-deepen the groove, as this may compromise bone strength and increase the risk of anchor pullout or inadequate fixation. The groove should be just deep enough to stabilize the tendon securely while preserving the structural integrity of the surrounding bone (**Figure 1B**).

5.2.5 Fixation and rerouting of LHBT

Fixation of LHBT is the central step of the SCR procedure. A suture anchor is inserted at the lateral edge of the neo-groove, and the tendon is secured using an onlay tenodesis technique, comparable to those commonly used in subpectoral biceps tenodesis. The arm should be positioned in approximately 30° to 45° of abduction during fixation to replicate the physiological tensioning typically applied in SCR. Tension must be optimized—tight enough to prevent tendon sagging, while allowing unrestricted passive shoulder range of motion. Although medial fixation of the tendon is technically possible, it is generally avoided due to concerns regarding vascular compromise. Excessive compression at the medial aspect may restrict blood flow to the tendon, impairing graft viability and healing. Instead, medial stabilization is achieved by approximating the remaining rotator cuff tissue over the rerouted LHBT, allowing the native cuff to function as a biological retainer without risking ischemia (**Figure 1C**).

5.2.6 Repair of the remaining rotator cuff

After fixation of LHBT, attention is directed to the remaining rotator cuff tissue. In most cases, a medially based single-row repair is preferred due to its lower tension profile; however, this may be tailored depending on the remaining tendon quality and mobility. Suture anchors are placed anterior and posterior to the rerouted LHBT along the medial footprint of the greater tuberosity. Sutures are then passed through the residual supraspinatus and infraspinatus tendons, followed by knot tying to complete a single-row construct. This configuration allows the repaired cuff to compress the LHBT against the greater tuberosity, thereby enhancing graft stability and promoting biologic healing. The biomechanical benefits of this approach include a substantial reduction in repair-site tension and the creation of a biologically favorable compression mechanism that stabilizes the LHBT graft (**Figure 1D** and **E**) Additional procedures may be performed based on intraoperative findings. Margin convergence can be utilized to approximate remaining rotator cuff tissue through side-to-side repair. Subacromial decompression, including limited acromioplasty, may be warranted in the presence of significant mechanical impingement. Finally, distal management of the LHBT can be adjusted based on surgeon preference and patient-specific factors. In some cases, the tendon is rerouted proximally for SCR while its distal portion is left untouched, with no tenotomy or tenodesis performed. Alternatively, the tendon can be transected just distal to its fixation point on the greater tuberosity, followed by tenodesis using an interference screw or suture anchor to minimize the risk of distal migration, muscle cramping, or cosmetic deformity.

5.3 Postoperative protocol

Postoperative rehabilitation following LHBT-SCR is designed to protect the graft while minimizing the risk of shoulder stiffness. In the early postoperative period, typically the first 6 weeks, the shoulder is immobilized in a sling to allow for initial healing. During this time, only limited passive range of motion is permitted, with gradual increases as tolerated. Rehabilitation exercises focus on pendulum movements, gentle passive stretching, and scapular stabilization. Patients must avoid active shoulder elevation, lifting, and any contraction of the biceps to prevent undue stress on the repair construct. After sling discontinuation, typically beginning at 6 weeks, the patient transitions to active range of motion exercises in all planes. Light strengthening of the remaining rotator cuff muscles is initiated while continuing to restrict any biceps loading or heavy lifting. From 12 weeks onward, the rehabilitation protocol progresses to a strengthening phase, during which full active range of motion is maintained through ongoing stretching. Progressive resistance training is introduced for the rotator cuff, and if the distal biceps tendon was preserved, light biceps strengthening may begin. Overhead lifting of more than 10 pounds should still be avoided until at least 16 weeks postoperatively to reduce stress on the reconstruction site. Beyond 20 weeks, patients begin activity-specific or sport-specific training. Light recreational activities are generally permitted for 4 to 5 months, with a full return to non-contact sports around 6 months. For those involved in contact sports or physically demanding occupations, return to full activity is typically delayed until 6 to 9 months postoperatively, based on individual recovery and functional readiness.

5.4 Tips and pitfalls

Optimal tension management is essential during LHBT-SCR. Excessive tension can limit shoulder mobility, while insufficient tension may lead to persistent superior migration of the humeral head. The graft should be tensioned adequately to prevent sagging while allowing full passive motion. Tension should be assessed arthroscopically by observing the behavior of the graft during manipulation of the joint. Throughout the procedure, care must be taken to minimize graft handling with instruments to avoid mechanical damage. When preparing the neo-groove on the lateral aspect of the greater tuberosity, care must be taken not to over-deepen it, as this may compromise bone integrity and reduce the security of fixation. Anchors should be appropriately sized according to the patient's bone quality, and their stability should be confirmed before graft fixation to ensure reliable mechanical support. Additionally, if intraoperative assessment reveals inadequate LHBT quality, the surgeon must be prepared with a backup plan, including the use of an allograft or partial rotator cuff repair. Repair of the remaining rotator cuff tendon is strongly recommended, as it enhances the stability of the construct, provides additional biological coverage over the graft, and facilitates healing. The subscapularis tendon, in particular, should not be overlooked, as its integrity is critical for maintaining anterior-posterior force coupling. Even when other portions of the cuff are irreparable, proper restoration of the subscapularis is essential for preserving shoulder mechanics and achieving favorable clinical outcomes. Postoperative rehabilitation should be customized based on intraoperative assessment of tissue quality and the overall security of graft fixation to optimize recovery and functional outcomes.

6. Conclusion and clinical implications

LHBT-SCR offers a practical, biologically favorable, and cost-effective solution for managing massive, irreparable posterosuperior RCTs. This technique utilizes autologous tissue readily available within the surgical field, thereby eliminating the need for allograft or additional donor site morbidity. Biomechanically, the LHBT provides sufficient integrity to support the joint's stabilizing architecture while preserving kinematics. When used as a pedicled graft, its preserved vascularity may promote biologic incorporation and enhance healing potential.

Early clinical results have demonstrated meaningful improvements in pain relief, range of motion, and functional scores—outcomes that are often comparable to those achieved with more complex or costly reconstruction techniques. However, the success of LHBT-SCR depends critically on proper patient selection, particularly in ensuring the presence of an intact subscapularis tendon and structurally viable LHBT tissue. Notably, grafts with partial tearing greater than 50% have been associated with inferior outcomes, highlighting the importance of careful intraoperative assessment.

The evolving role of LHBT-SCR reflects a broader paradigm shift toward biologically sound, joint-preserving approaches in shoulder reconstruction. Future prospective trials should prioritize stratifying outcomes by tendon integrity, tear configuration, and subscapularis status, while also evaluating long-term cost-effectiveness and durability in diverse healthcare settings.

Author details

Kyun-Ho Shin[1]*, Seung-Beom Han[2] and Il-Tae Jang[3]

1 Department of Orthopedic Surgery, Juan Nanoori Hospital, Incheon, Republic of Korea

2 Department of Orthopedic Surgery, Korea University Anam Hospital, Seoul, Republic of Korea

3 Nanoori Medical Research Institute, Seoul, Republic of Korea

*Address all correspondence to: kyunho.shin@gmail.com

References

[1] Burkhart SS, Danaceau SM, Pearce CE Jr. Arthroscopic rotator cuff repair: Analysis of results by tear size and by repair technique—Margin convergence versus direct tendon-to-bone repair. Arthroscopy. 2001;**17**(9):905-912. DOI: 10.1053/jars.2001.28181

[2] Lo IK, Burkhart SS. Arthroscopic repair of massive, contracted, immobile rotator cuff tears using single and double interval slides: Technique and preliminary results. Arthroscopy. 2004;**20**(1):22-33. DOI: 10.1016/j.arthro.2003.11.005

[3] Favard L, Berhouet J, Colmar M, Boukobza E, Richou J, Sonnard A, et al. Massive rotator cuff tears in patients younger than 65 years. What treatment options are available. Orthopaedics & Traumatology, Surgery & Research. 2009;**95**(4):19-26. DOI: 10.1016/J.OTSR.2009.03.005

[4] Muench LN, Dyrna F, Beitzel K. Massive and irreparable rotator cuff tears: Defining the problem. In: Massive and Irreparable Rotator Cuff Tears. Berlin, Heidelberg: Springer; 2020. pp. 3-10. DOI: 10.1007/978-3-662-61162-3_1

[5] Di Benedetto P, Mancuso F, Tosolini L, Buttironi MM, Beltrame A, Causero A. Treatment options for massive rotator cuff tears: A narrative review. Acta Bio-Medica. 2021;**92**(S3):e2021026. DOI: 10.23750/ABM.V92IS3.11766

[6] Galatz LM, Ball CM, Teefey SA, Middleton WD, Yamaguchi K. The outcome and repair integrity of completely arthroscopically repaired large and massive rotator cuff tears. The Journal of Bone and Joint Surgery. American Volume. 2004;**86**(2):219-224. DOI: 10.2106/00004623-200402000-00001

[7] Boileau P, Brassart N, Watkinson DJ, Carles M, Hatzidakis AM, Krishnan SG. Arthroscopic repair of full-thickness tears of the supraspinatus: Does the tendon really heal? The Journal of Bone and Joint Surgery. American Volume. 2005;**87**(6):1229-1240. DOI: 10.2106/JBJS.D.02035

[8] Hansen M, Otis JC, Johnson JS, Cordasco FA, Craig EV, Warren RF. Biomechanics of massive rotator cuff tears: Implications for treatment. The Journal of Bone and Joint Surgery. American Volume. 2008;**90**(2):316-325. DOI: 10.2106/JBJS.F.00880

[9] Woodmass JM, Wagner ER, Chang MJ, Welp KM, Elhassan BT, Higgins LD, et al. Arthroscopic treatment of massive posterosuperior rotator cuff tears: A critical analysis review. JBJS Reviews. 2018;**6**(9):e4. DOI: 10.2106/JBJS.RVW.17.00199

[10] Denard PJ. An algorithmic approach to the surgical management of massive rotator cuff tears based on imaging, function, and repairability. Arthroscopy. 2023;**39**(11):2392-2397. DOI: 10.1016/j.arthro.2023.06.017

[11] Mulieri PJ, Dunning P, Klein SM, Pupello D, Frankle MA. Reverse shoulder arthroplasty for the treatment of irreparable rotator cuff tear without glenohumeral arthritis. The Journal of Bone and Joint Surgery. American Volume. 2010;**92**(15):2544-2556. DOI: 10.2106/JBJS.I.00912

[12] Ernstbrunner L, Suter A, Catanzaro S, Rahm S, Gerber C. Reverse total shoulder arthroplasty for massive,

irreparable rotator cuff tears before the age of 60 years: Long-term results. The Journal of Bone and Joint Surgery. American Volume. 2017;**99**(20):1721-1729. DOI: 10.2106/JBJS.17.00095

[13] Viswanath A, Bale S, Trail I. Reverse total shoulder arthroplasty for irreparable rotator cuff tears without arthritis: A systematic review. Journal of Clinical Orthopaedics and Trauma. 2021;**17**:267-272. DOI: 10.1016/j.jcot.2021.04.005

[14] Morgan WA. Reverse total shoulder arthroplasty for younger patients: A comparable analysis of patients older and younger than 65 years. JAAOS Global Research & Reviews. 2023;**7**(6):e23.00064. DOI: 10.5435/jaaosglobal-d-22-00264

[15] Mihata T, McGarry MH, Pirolo JM, Kinoshita M, Lee TQ. Superior capsule reconstruction to restore superior stability in irreparable rotator cuff tears: A biomechanical cadaveric study. The American Journal of Sports Medicine. 2012;**40**(10):2248-2255. DOI: 10.1177/0363546512456195

[16] Mihata T, Lee TQ, Watanabe C, Fukunishi K, Ohue M, Tsujimura T, et al. Clinical results of arthroscopic superior capsule reconstruction for irreparable rotator cuff tears. Arthroscopy. 2013;**29**(3):459-470. DOI: 10.1016/j.arthro.2012.10.002

[17] Mihata T, Bui CNH, Akeda M, Cavagnaro MA, Kuenzler M, Peterson AB, et al. A biomechanical cadaveric study comparing superior capsule reconstruction using fascia lata allograft with human dermal allograft for irreparable rotator cuff tear. Journal of Shoulder and Elbow Surgery. 2017;**26**(12):2158-2166. DOI: 10.1016/j.jse.2017.07.019

[18] Pennington WT, Bartz BA, Pauli JM, Walker CE, Schmidt W. Arthroscopic superior capsular reconstruction with acellular dermal allograft for the treatment of massive irreparable rotator cuff tears: Short-term clinical outcomes and the radiographic parameter of superior capsular distance. Arthroscopy. 2018;**34**(6):1764-1773. DOI: 10.1016/j.arthro.2018.01.009

[19] Woodmass J, Wagner E, Borque K, Chang M, Welp K, Warner J. Superior capsule reconstruction using dermal allograft: Early outcomes and survival. Journal of Shoulder and Elbow Surgery. 2019;**28**(6S):S100-S109. DOI: 10.1016/j.jse.2019.04.011

[20] Burkhart SS, Hartzler RU. Superior capsular reconstruction reverses profound pseudoparalysis in patients with irreparable rotator cuff tears and minimal or no glenohumeral arthritis. Arthroscopy. 2019;**35**(1):22-28. DOI: 10.1016/j.arthro.2018.06.032

[21] Lacheta L, Horan MP, Schairer WW, Goldenberg BT, Dornan GJ, Pogorzelski J, et al. Clinical and imaging outcomes after arthroscopic superior capsule reconstruction with human dermal allograft for irreparable posterosuperior rotator cuff tears: A minimum 2-year follow-up. Arthroscopy. 2020;**36**(4):1011-1019. DOI: 10.1016/j.arthro.2019.12.024

[22] Burkhart SS, Pranckun JJ, Hartzler RU. Superior capsular reconstruction for the operatively irreparable rotator cuff tear: Clinical outcomes are maintained 2 years after surgery. Arthroscopy. 2020;**36**(2):373-380. DOI: 10.1016/j.arthro.2019.08.035

[23] Takayama K, Ito H. Clinical effectiveness of superior capsular reconstruction using Teflon felt graft in the elderly for pain relief: A comparison using tensor fascia lata graft. JSES International. 2023;**7**(6):2379-2388. DOI: 10.1016/j.jseint.2023.07.006

[24] El-Shaar R, Soin S, Nicandri G, Maloney M, Voloshin I. Superior capsular reconstruction with a long head of the biceps tendon autograft: A cadaveric study. Orthopaedic Journal of Sports Medicine. 2018;**6**(7):2325967118785365. DOI: 10.1177/2325967118785365

[25] Rhee SM, Youn SM, Park JH, Rhee YG. Biceps rerouting for semirigid large-to-massive rotator cuff tears. Arthroscopy. 2021;**37**(9):2769-2779. DOI: 10.1016/j.arthro.2021.03.037

[26] McClatchy SG, Parsell DE, Hobgood ER, Field LD. Augmentation of massive rotator cuff repairs using biceps transposition without tenotomy improves clinical and patient-reported outcomes: The biological superior capsular reconstruction technique. Arthroscopy. 2023;**40**(1):47-54. DOI: 10.1016/j.arthro.2022.07.010

[27] Millett PJ, Warth RJ, Dornan GJ, Lee JT, Spiegl UJA. Massive rotator cuff tears: Pathomechanics, current treatment options, and clinical outcomes. Journal of Shoulder and Elbow Surgery. 2014;**23**(12):188-202. DOI: 10.1016/j.jse.2014.08.001

[28] Thomas K, Kendal JK, Ono Y, Lo IKY, Bois AJ. The role of partial rotator cuff repairs in patients with massive irreparable tears without arthritis. Orthopedics. 2020;**43**(1):1-6. DOI: 10.3928/01477447-20191031-05

[29] Ishigaki N, Hata Y, Matsuba T, Hino M, Murakami N, Kobayashi H. Long-term results of partial repair for irreparable rotator cuff tear. JSES International. 2021;**5**(4):642-648. DOI: 10.1016/j.jseint.2021.02.010

[30] Iannotti JP, Hennigan S, Herzog R, Kella S, Kelley M, Leggin B, et al. Latissimus dorsi tendon transfer for irreparable posterosuperior rotator cuff tears: Factors affecting outcome. The Journal of Bone and Joint Surgery. American Volume. 2006;**88**(2):342-348. DOI: 10.2106/JBJS.D.02996

[31] Galasso O, Mantovani M, Muraccini M, et al. The latissimus dorsi tendon functions as an external rotator after arthroscopic-assisted transfer for massive irreparable posterosuperior rotator cuff tears. Knee Surgery, Sports Traumatology, Arthroscopy. 2020;**28**:2367-2376. DOI: 10.1007/s00167-019-05819-2

[32] Waltenspül M, Jochum B, Filli L, Ernstbrunner L, Wieser K, Meyer DC, et al. Mid-term results of arthroscopically assisted latissimus dorsi transfer for irreparable posterosuperior rotator cuff tears. Journal of Shoulder and Elbow Surgery. 2021;**30**(11):e676-e688. DOI: 10.1016/j.jse.2021.03.149

[33] Gavriilidis I, Kircher J, Magosch P, Lichtenberg S, Habermeyer P. Pectoralis major transfer for the treatment of irreparable anterosuperior rotator cuff tears. International Orthopaedics. 2010;**34**(5):689-694. DOI: 10.1007/s00264-009-0799-9

[34] Shin JJ, Saccomanno MF, Cole BJ, Romeo AA, Nicholson GP, Verma NN. Pectoralis major transfer for treatment of irreparable subscapularis tear: A systematic review. Knee Surgery, Sports Traumatology, Arthroscopy. 2016;**24**(6):1951-1960. DOI: 10.1007/s00167-014-3229-5

[35] de Marinis R, Marigi EM, Atwan Y, Velasquez Garcia A, Morrey ME, Sanchez-Sotelo J. Lower trapezius transfer improves clinical outcomes with a rate of complications and reoperations comparable to other surgical alternatives in patients with functionally irreparable rotator cuff tears: A systematic review. Arthroscopy.

2024;**40**(3):950-959. DOI: 10.1016/j.arthro.2023.06.029

[36] Choi S, Kim G, Lee Y, et al. Patch augmentation does not provide better clinical outcomes than arthroscopic rotator cuff repair for large to massive rotator cuff tears. Knee Surgery, Sports Traumatology, Arthroscopy. 2022;**30**:3851-3861. DOI: 10.1007/s00167-022-06975-8

[37] Kim KT, Kim GH, Cha DH, Lee JH, Lee YB. A comparison of clinical outcomes in rotator cuff re-tear patients who had either an arthroscopic primary repair or arthroscopic patch augmentation for large-to-massive rotator cuff tears. Diagnostics (Basel). 2023;**13**(11):1961. DOI: 10.3390/diagnostics13111961

[38] Lederman ES, Toth AP, Nicholson GP, Nowinski RJ, Bal GK, Williams GR, et al. A prospective, multicenter study to evaluate clinical and radiographic outcomes in primary rotator cuff repair reinforced with a xenograft dermal matrix. Journal of Shoulder and Elbow Surgery. 2016;**25**(12):1961-1970. DOI: 10.1016/j.jse.2016.02.029

[39] Ciampi P, Scotti C, Nonis A, Vitali M, Di Serio C, Peretti GM, et al. The benefit of synthetic versus biological patch augmentation in the repair of posterosuperior massive rotator cuff tears: A 3-year follow-up study. The American Journal of Sports Medicine. 2014;**42**(5):1169-1175. DOI: 10.1177/0363546514525592

[40] Gomes N, Fonte H, Santos S, Sousa D. Subacromial resurfacing with fascia lata autograft for irreparable cuff tears: JEO 2021 expert opinion short report & surgical technique with video. Journal of Experimental Orthopaedics. 2021;**8**:64. DOI: 10.1186/s40634-021-00364-2

[41] Smith TJ, Gowd AK, Kunkel J, Kaplin L, Waterman BR. Superior capsular reconstruction provides sufficient biomechanical outcomes for massive, irreparable rotator cuff tears: A systematic review. Arthroscopy. 2021;**37**(1):402-410. DOI: 10.1016/j.arthro.2020.09.007

[42] Cohn M, Vadhera A, Garrigues G, Verma N. Superior capsular reconstruction: Proposed biomechanical advantages. Arthroscopy. 2022;**38**(1):20-21. DOI: 10.1016/j.arthro.2021.11.011

[43] Shin KH, Jang IT, Han SB. Outcomes of superior capsular reconstruction using the long head of the biceps tendon in large to massive rotator cuff tears: A meta-analysis and systematic review. Journal of Clinical Medicine. 2024;**13**(4):1052. DOI: 10.3390/jcm13041052

[44] Kholinne E, Kwak JM, Kim H, Koh KH, Jeon IH. Arthroscopic superior capsular reconstruction with mesh augmentation for the treatment of irreparable rotator cuff tears: A comparative study of surgical outcomes. The American Journal of Sports Medicine. 2020;**48**(13):3328-3338. DOI: 10.1177/0363546520958708

[45] Bi M, Ding W, Zheng M, Peng Z, Li J, Ding S. Arthroscopic superior capsule reconstruction with combined fascia lata autograft and synthetic scaffold patch graft for the treatment of irreparable rotator cuff tears yields favorable clinical and radiographic outcomes at minimum 2-year follow-up. Arthroscopy. 2023;**39**(8):1800-1810. DOI: 10.1016/j.arthro.2023.02.025

[46] Da Silva AZ, Mizels J, Clinker CE, Yoo M, Nelson R, Joyce C, et al. Cost analysis of dermal allograft patch utilization in rotator cuff repair. JSES Reviews, Reports and Techniques.

2024;**5**(1):40-45. DOI: 10.1016/j.xrrt.2024.08.011

[47] Candela V, Preziosi Standoli J, Carbone S, Rionero M, Gumina S. Shoulder long head biceps tendon pathology is associated with increasing rotator cuff tear size. Arthroscopy, Sports Medicine, and Rehabilitation. 2021;**3**(5):e1517-e1523. DOI: 10.1016/j.asmr.2021.07.013

[48] Han F, Kong CH, Hasan MY, Ramruttun AK, Kumar VP. Superior capsular reconstruction for irreparable supraspinatus tendon tears using the long head of biceps: A biomechanical study on cadavers. Orthopaedics & Traumatology, Surgery & Research. 2019;**105**(2):257-263. DOI: 10.1016/j.otsr.2018.10.023

[49] Chiang CH, Shaw L, Chih WH, Yeh ML, Ting HH, Lin CH, et al. Modified superior capsule reconstruction using the long head of the biceps tendon as reinforcement to rotator cuff repair lowers retear rate in large to massive reparable rotator cuff tears. Arthroscopy. 2021;**37**(8):2420-2431. DOI: 10.1016/j.arthro.2021.04.003

[50] Barth J, Olmos MI, Swan J, Barthelemy R, Delsol P, Boutsiadis A. Superior capsular reconstruction with the long head of the biceps autograft prevents infraspinatus retear in massive posterosuperior retracted rotator cuff tears. The American Journal of Sports Medicine. 2020;**48**(6):1430-1438. DOI: 10.1177/0363546520912220

[51] Llinás PJ, Bailie DS, Sanchez DA, Chica J, Londoño JF, Herrera GA. Partial superior capsular reconstruction to augment arthroscopic repair of massive rotator cuff tears using autogenous biceps tendon: Effect on retear rate. The American Journal of Sports Medicine. 2022;**50**(11):3064-3072. DOI: 10.1177/03635465221112659

[52] Kawashima K, Terabayashi N, Asano H, Akiyama H. Arthroscopic long head of the biceps transposition for superior capsular augmentation results in comparable clinical outcomes to arthroscopic partial repair for irreparable rotator cuff tears. Arthroscopy, Sports Medicine, and Rehabilitation. 2022;**4**(5):e425-e434. DOI: 10.1016/j.asmr.2022.04.003

Chapter 8

Shoulder Arthroplasty in the Active Athlete

Neal Krentz, Benjamin Sanderford, Kelly Wolfe and Andrew Ames

Abstract

Total shoulder arthroplasty (TSA) is an effective treatment option for a broad spectrum of shoulder pathologies ranging from arthritis, osteonecrosis, fracture or rotator cuff dysfunction. Patients consenting to TSA are seeking improvement in shoulder pain, function and desire to maintain an active lifestyle. The level of activity in patients undergoing TSA varies significantly; from the patient who wishes to be able to garden to the patient who wishes to continue competitive weightlifting. While return to sport following total hip and total knee arthroplasty is more established, less evidence exists surrounding TSA. Return to sport rates are promising for anatomic total shoulder arthroplasty (aTSA), being reported as high as 75–100%. This rate however may vary significantly based on the sport and patient. Return to sport rates vary between aTSA, hemiarthroplasty (HA) and reverse total shoulder arthroplasty (rTSA). While most surgeons allow return to low-impact activities such as swimming, biking, or golf, there is less agreement in return to higher impact activities such as contact sports, rowing or weightlifting. Higher impact sports place more mechanical stress across the rotator cuff and prosthesis, placing patients at a higher risk for complications. Regardless, surgeons agree that return to sport following TSA is within the realm of possibility and individualized treatment plans should be tailored for each patient.

Keywords: return to sport, glenohumeral arthritis, total shoulder arthroplasty, athlete, weightlifter, post-operative restrictions

1. Introduction

The incidence of total shoulder arthroplasty (TSA) is rising in the United States as patients seek options to treat painful shoulder arthritis and maintain healthy, active lifestyles [1–9]. Shoulder arthroplasty implants are now in their fourth generation with widespread reported good to excellent results achievable after surgery. Patients undergoing TSA seek pain relief and functional improvement. As outcomes continue to improve, so too do patient's expectations after surgery. Many patients now wish to return to sport (RTS) following TSA, which has been reported to be as high as 64% of patients [10].

Return to sport is a significant outcome for a subset of active patients. Studies have demonstrated that most patients can expect to RTS, and that greater than 70% of patients can return at an equal or improved level of competition [4]. However, these numbers historically have been tied to more elderly patients participating in lower intensity sports, such as golf or cycling, and patient satisfaction is less predictable in younger, more active patients, despite similar functional outcomes and high rates of RTS [1]. A paucity of literature exists regarding outcomes in specific cohorts with very high demand athletic activity, such as weightlifters.

Surgeons' restrictions vary for return to sports following shoulder arthroplasty. Surgeons have been unable to reach a consensus for recommendations on return to multiple sports including baseball/softball, lacrosse, rowing, soccer, and weightlifting [6]. A survey of international surgeons was conducted, and revealed that 57% recommended against weightlifting after anatomic TSA, and 82% recommended against lifting following reverse TSA [7]. Against surgeon recommendations, high-level postoperative athletic activity, including weightlifting, has been described [3, 11–14].

The ideal surgery for the younger, active patient with glenohumeral arthritis and an intact rotator cuff has been a debate for decades. Hemiarthroplasty (HA) was once viewed as the safer option, as glenoid loosening leading to difficult and lesser outcome revision surgery was a feared complication of aTSA. However recent evidence suggests this historical dogma no longer applies. While both surgeries have proven to create significant improvements in pain and function from preoperative levels, comparatively patients have experienced improved satisfaction and return to sport rates following aTSA [1, 3]. Additional studies have eluded to improved longevity, lower revision rates [15] and lower overall cost [16] following TSA versus HA. Although glenoid loosening remains the leading cause of revision total shoulder arthroplasty [17], the overall reported rate remains low (1.9% of aTSA) and [3, 10, 11, 14, 18, 19] medium-term studies and meta-analyses [1, 2, 4, 8, 15] have shown little to no glenoid failure even in more active patients. The most modern implants have been designed with new strategies to reduce glenoid loosening through a partial inlay design.

This chapter will present the current literature around overall return to sport rates following TSA with a focus on aTSA, sport specific evidence and expert opinion, return to sport rates between the different kinds of TSA (aTSA), HA and reverse total shoulder arthroplasty (rTSA) and briefly discuss glenoid loosening as it relates to return to sport.

2. Return to sport following total shoulder arthroplasty

Shoulder arthroplasty, including Anatomic Total Shoulder Arthroplasty (aTSA), Reverse Total Shoulder Arthroplasty (rTSA), and Hemiarthroplasty (HA), aims at alleviating pain and restoring function in patients with severe shoulder joint pathology. The indications for the procedure (i.e. arthritis, fracture, tumor, etc.), type of shoulder arthroplasty performed, the patient's preoperative activity levels, and the specific demands of the sport play crucial roles in determining the likelihood and timeline for returning to sports. Both HA and aTSA are indicated in patients with shoulder osteoarthritis and intact rotator cuff function. Surgeons have expressed confidence in allowing patients to return from sport following both aTSA and HA, and with less confidence rTSA [5–7]. Both provide pain relief and a relatively high rate of RTS. For many patients undergoing TSA, the ability to return to sports and recreational activities post-surgery is a significant concern [10]. Return to sport rates are multifactorial and depend on patient age, prior activity level, which sports they wish to return to and surgeon comfort in allowing return to said sport. There is no one-size-fits-all approach, and it is in the best interest of the patient and surgeon to provide full disclosure and realistic expectations prior to undergoing a major procedure like TSA.

2.1 Rehabilitation protocols

Returning to sport following TSA is a gradual, patient-specific process that begins with a structured rehabilitation protocol requiring a collaborative effort between the surgeon and physical therapists. Multiple different rehab protocols published by multiple institutions are available online, however significant variance [20] occurs between these protocols. A consensus currently does not exist on the timing of initiation of physical therapy following TSA. The American Society of Shoulder and Elbow Therapists (ASSET) produced a set of recommendation guidelines following aTSA based on three 6-week intervals which are summarized later in this section [21].

Operative factors including implant selection, the quality of bone stock, the management and quality of repair of the subscapularis and biceps tendon may contribute to variance in rehabilitation protocols. Communication between the surgeon, patient and physical therapist throughout the rehab process is crucial for successful recovery. Overprotection may lead to stiffness while overly aggressive protocols may compromise healing and result in poor outcomes. This specifically applies to external rotation (ER). Although no differences in clinical outcomes have been demonstrated between subscapularis peel, tenotomy and lesser tuberosity osteotomy [22], surgeon-specific protocols to allow for healing may differ and should be communicated.

Phase 1 of the ASSET guidelines encompasses the immediate post-op period from post-op day #1 to post-op week #6. This phase focuses on pain control, protection of the implant and allowing for the healing of soft tissues. Patients should remain non-weightbearing in the operative extremity. Patients should avoid active motion of the glenohumeral joint, while active scapular retraction and active motion of the elbow and wrist are permitted. Patients should remain immobilized in a sling or shoulder immobilizer with an abduction pillow 24/7, only to remove for home exercises and hygiene. 59% of surgeons surveyed recommended 4 weeks of immobilization, while 24% recommended 6 weeks. The minority recommended 2 weeks or no sling at all [21]. Home exercises consist of pendulum exercises (**Figure 1**) and passive range of motion (PROM) in forward flexion and ER. While specific limits vary, the ASSET guidelines recommend limiting forward flexion to 120° and external rotation to 30° [18]. Non-impact activities such as walking or stationary biking are permitted once the incision has healed. Patients may progress to Phase 2 once their incision is healed, pain is well controlled and cleared by their surgeon.

Phase 2 occurs from 4 to 6 weeks post-op until 12 weeks post-op and centers around optimizing PROM, developing active range of motion (AROM) and strengthening the periscapular muscles, rotator cuff and deltoid through AROM exercises against gravity only (**Figure 2**). Once PROM goals are met, patients are encouraged to begin AROM with forward flexion, ER and internal rotation (IR). ER and IR exercises are performed in the seated and side lying positions. ER and IR exercises are begun with the shoulder adducted against the body with gradual progression of shoulder abduction to 90°. Scapular protraction and retraction exercises against gravity are permitted. Aerobic activities and lower body weight training are allowed in this phase so long as no upper extremity resistance is involved (i.e. using the arm on an elliptical

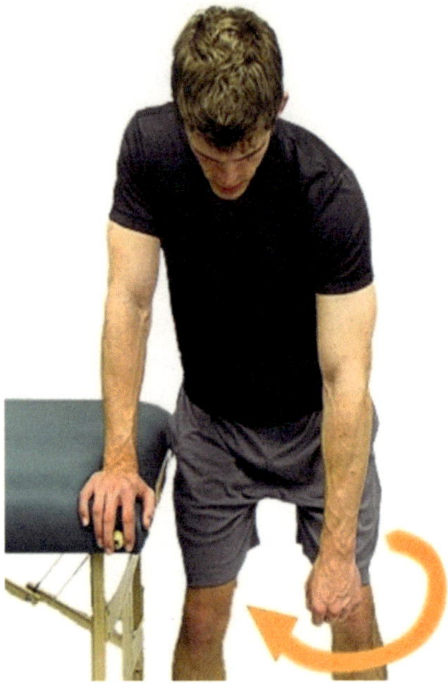

Figure 1.
Pendulum exercises to be performed in phase 1 of rehab.

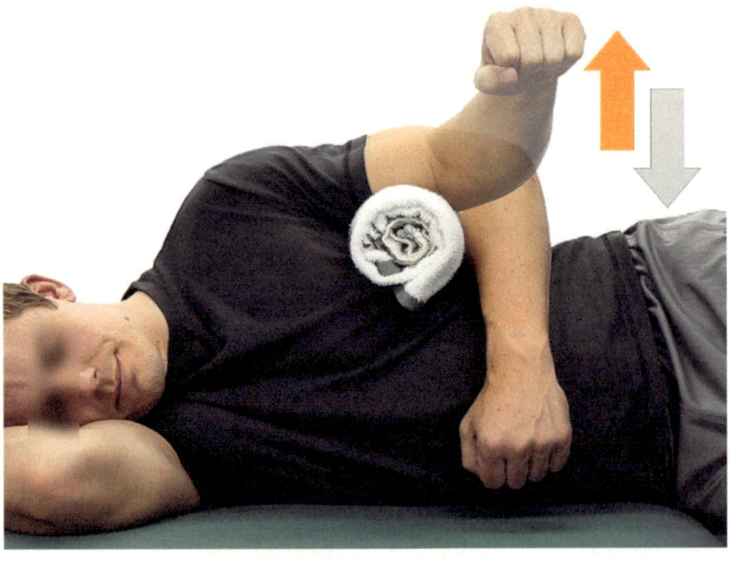

Figure 2.
External and internal rotation exercises against gravity.

machine). Patients progress to Phase 3 once pain-free AROM against gravity equals PROM and both patients and surgeons are comfortable with progressing to higher levels of activity beyond activities of daily living.

Phase 3 generally begins at 12 weeks post-op and centers around strengthening, patient and sport specific demands. The goals of this phase are to gradually increase strength of the deltoid, rotator cuff, biceps and periscapular muscles leading to functional mobility and pain-free use of the shoulder. Exercises employed in this phase include gentle stretching, strengthening with light resistance such as bands (**Figure 3**), weights and machines. Shoulder specific exercises are kept in the anterior and frontal plane. Overhead exercises should be avoided. Closed chain exercises such as planks may be resumed. Return to low-impact sports may be introduced in this time period. This includes golf, swimming and jogging. However this should be introduced slowly and full return to sport should be cautioned. Higher-load activities such as bench press should be avoided until at least 6 months.

While return to sport is promising in patients undergoing TSA, most experts would agree that return to full participation should be avoided until 3–6 months at the earliest [5–7]. Following a structured rehab protocol and obtaining clearance by the performing surgeon should be undertaken prior to return to sport.

2.2 Low-impact sports

Low impact sports include golf, bowling, rowing, cycling, swimming, yoga, and running. Surgeons can feel confident allowing their patients to return following TSA. Surveys conducted amongst orthopedic surgeons have concluded that the majority are comfortable allowing patients to return to low-impact sports following aTSA. In a survey of 94 surgeons >80% said they would allow their patients to return to sport with golf, cycling, swimming and yoga being allowed by >90% of respondents [5]. Patients may begin sport-specific exercises as early as 3 months postoperatively in most scenarios, but patients should be educated that full return to sport may not occur until 6–12 months [2, 18].

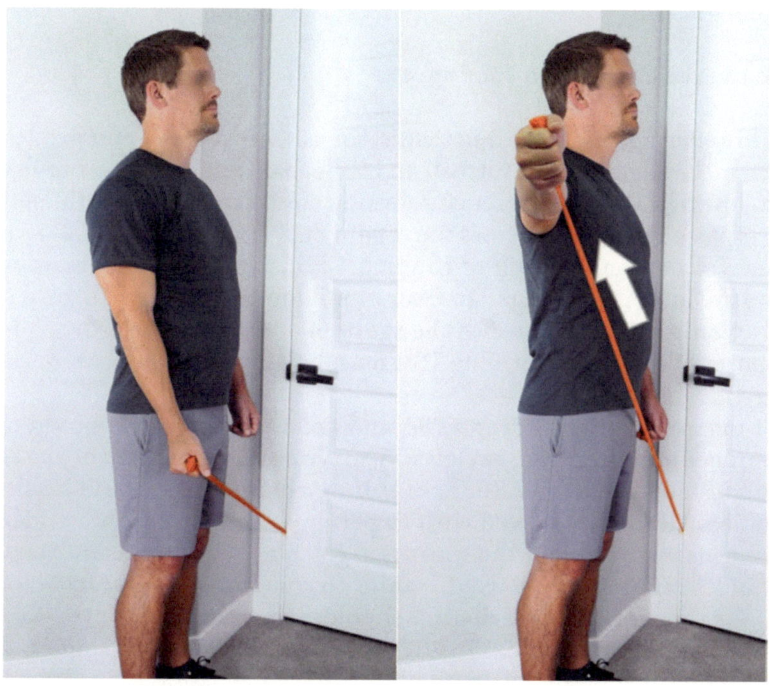

Figure 3.
Light resistance band exercises to begin strengthening.

Overall, return to full participation in low-impact sports is promising following aTSA with 75–100% of patients returning to sport [2–4, 10, 18]. Historically, the majority of patients who undergo aTSA are able to return to low impact sports at a similar or even improved level of play. Jensen et al. [23] followed 23 patients who wished to return to golf following shoulder arthroplasty (20 aTSA and 6 HA). Average time to return to playing a full round of golf was 4.5 months and 18 patients were able to improve by 5 strokes compared to their preoperative handicap. McCarty et al. [10] reviewed a case series of return to sport in patients who underwent aTSA and HA. Of the aTSA cohort, 44 of 54 (81.5%) returned to sport. They noted a 92% return to fishing, 86% return to swimming, 75% return to golf and 60% return to rowing/kayaking. Average time to partial return was 3.6 months and full return was 5.8 months. Days active increased from 0.7 to 1.7 days from pre to post-op. Bulhoff et al. [19] reviewed 87 patients (mean age 71 years old, mean follow-up 6.2 years) who were participating in sports within 5 years of their aTSA. The most popular sports in their cohort were swimming, tennis, fitness activities and golf. They found 90% of patients in this cohort returned to sport. This number increased to 100% in the 57 patients who were active in their sport immediately prior to their aTSA. Schumann et al. [24] reported 89% (49 of 55) patients were able to resume playing sports at an average follow-up of 2.8 years, however 36.7% were limited by their shoulder. Of note, a significant improvement in performance was noted by the golfer cohort in their study.

Return to low demand sports following aTSA appears promising. Increased chance of return to full sport is seen in patients who have a higher level of function prior to surgery, higher levels of motivation to return to sport, and adhere to their post-operative rehab protocols. Although a return to low-impact sports is likely following aTSA, surgeons must counsel their patients that return to an equal or improved level of sport is not guaranteed.

2.3 Racket, overhead and high-load sports

Return to racket sports, including tennis, squash, racquetball and pickleball, overhead sports, including baseball, softball and volleyball, and high-load sports like rock climbing following aTSA presents an interesting clinical problem for the surgeons. These sports place more stress across the rotator cuff and prosthesis and require greater ranges of motion than golf or running. Racket sports offer numerous health benefits and are increasingly popular. Over 21 million people participate in racket sports and an estimated 37% are over the age of 60 [14]. With the growing interest in racket sports, surgeons performing TSA must be prepared to answer questions regarding return to play.

Most of the evidence regarding aTSA and racket sports is composed of Level IV or V evidence and literature reviews. A survey of 35 members of the American Shoulder and Elbow Society (ASES) regarding which sports would be either Recommended/Allowed, Allowed with Experience, or Not Recommended. If <79% consensus was reached, the sport was given a "No Conclusion" recommendation. Doubles tennis was "allowed", while no conclusion was reached on singles tennis [6]. A survey of 101 experienced shoulder surgeons (47 North America, 52 Europe, 1 Asia, 1 South America) in 2011 reached consensus on singles, doubles tennis and racquetball being "allowed with experience" following aTSA [7]. A survey of 94 members of the ASES in 2012 found that over 75% of responders would "allow" tennis, racquetball and squash following TSA [5]. Based on survey responses, it would appear that surgeons are becoming more comfortable with their patients participating in racket sports following aTSA.

Evidence presented from several case series following return to racket sports in patients following aTSA is primarily positive. Mannava et al. [18] performed a case series of patients attempting to return to sport following aTSA from 2005 to 2015. Of the 20 patients whose preferred activity was "tennis/racquetball, overhead sports", 50% were able to return to their previous level of competition, 28.6% reported to be below their previous level and 21.4% were unable to return to play. A case series conducted by McCarty et al. published in 2008 included 32 patients who wished to return to tennis, racquetball or squash and noted a 75% return to play rate in this group [10]. Garcia et al. [3] reported an 87.5% return to singles tennis and an 83.8% return to "high upper extremity sports" in their case series of patients less than 55 years old undergoing aTSA. Lastly, Vegas et al. [14] published a case series in 2023 of patients returning to racket sports following shoulder arthroplasty and concluded that 96% of their 26 aTSA patients were able to return to sport. Of these patients, 50% returned to play at 6 months and 81% returned by 1 year. This study also highlighted that surgery performed on the dominant arm may also play a factor in the return to sport performance following shoulder arthroplasty. While no significant statistical difference was noted, there was an increased percentage of patients who felt their overall performance "improved" following TSA on their dominant arm. These findings support that patients undergoing aTSA have a realistic chance at returning to racket sports with improvement in shoulder pain and function. However, additional recovery time prior to play may be required for additional strengthening of the rotator cuff.

The literature on return to other high load upper extremity sports such as baseball, softball, volleyball and rock climbing is sparse and mainly confined to survey studies and small samples within case series. The survey participants Healy et al. [6] gave softball, baseball and volleyball a "no consensus" ruling while stating return to rock climbing was "not allowed". Magnussen et al. [7] also assigned volleyball, baseball/softball an "undecided" ruling on return to play. Of note, the majority of European surgeons in this survey voted "would not allow" while more American surgeons leaned towards "allow with experience". The results from Golant et al. [5] were slightly more lenient towards baseball/softball (70% "allowed to return") than previous surveys, but remained consistent with prior surveys with uncertainty surrounding volleyball (58.9–64.5% allowed to return) and rock climbing (46.4%). Evidence from case series on throwing athletes following are limited. McCarty et al. [10] noted only 2 of 10 patients were able to return to softball following aTSA. More research is required in this area to establish a true return to play rate for baseball or softball. To the authors knowledge, no case series exists on return to rock climbing following aTSA.

2.4 High-impact, contact sports

High impact sports include football, lacrosse, hockey, basketball and martial arts. These activities carry a much higher risk of possible injury or prosthesis failure. Patients wishing to return to these activities need to be counseled extensively. Literature around return to these activities following aTSA is limited. Surveys completed by Healy et al. and Magnussen et al. [6, 7] agree that return to hockey or football following aTSA should "not be allowed" by the surgeon. The survey by Golant et al. [5] expressed similar concerns with 49.1% of responders stating they would "not allow" return to "contact sports" compared to only 8.2% that would "allow without restrictions" following aTSA. Basketball was viewed most favorably by the Golant survey respondents, with 74.2% allowing return in some capacity. The case series by Garcia et al. [3] echoed this sentiment with 75% (6 of 8) of patients ages less than 55 were able to return to play basketball. They concluded that "younger athletic patients can return to a larger number and higher demand of sports than has been previously described". Further research into outcomes in high-demand, younger patients undergoing aTSA is required before any consensus can be reached on the safety of return to contact sports.

2.5 Non-upper extremity sports with fall risk

Other sports yet to have been discussed are downhill skiing, snowboarding, horseback riding, soccer, ice skating which have been classified as non-upper extremity sports with high fall risks. Counseling patients on return to these sports following aTSA highlights the importance of approaching each patient's needs on an individual basis. For example, a patient who has never ice skated before and wishes to learn following aTSA carries a significantly high risk of injury compared to a seasoned hockey player who would like to skate recreationally. The literature on return following aTSA is again limited in these areas. In the opinions of shoulder surgeons, skiing, soccer and skating carry the lowest risk upon return to sport following aTSA. The respondents to the surveys conducted by Healy et al. and Magnussen et al. [6, 7] stated they would "allow to return with prior experience" for those wishing to pursue skiing and ice skating. The same respondents were "undecided" on snowboarding. The majority of responders to the survey by Golant et al. voted in favor of allowing return in some capacity to horseback riding (87.6%), ice skating (86.2%), skiing (81.2%), soccer (71.3%) and snowboarding (58.2%). Of the 28 patients in the "snow sports" subgroup of patients hoping to return to skiing, snowboarding and hockey in the case series by Mannava et al. [18], 56.2% were able to return to their prior level of activity, 43.8% were are to return to a lesser level of activity while 0% reported their were unable to return however this was not specific to any single sport. While confidence seems to grow with allowing experienced athletes to return to sport, surgeons may want to have a thorough discussion with patients about their prior level of activity, anticipated level of activity following aTSA and the inherent risks involved.

2.6 Weightlifting

Weightlifting finds a unique place amongst the sports that a patient may return to following aTSA. Weightlifting places repetitive, high loads across the glenohumeral joint. This elevates surgeon's concerns for glenoid component failure and accelerated component wear. The survey of international surgeons conducted by Magnussen et al. [7] revealed that 57% recommended against weightlifting after anatomic TSA. This is echoed by case series with "no heavy weightlifting" restrictions placed on patients following aTSA [3]. Studies investigating return to weightlifting have been vague with loose definitions including "fitness sports" or "resistance bands" and do not offer much insight into those who wish to resume more strenuous forms of weightlifting [25]. Recent literature has focused on high-demand weightlifters who represent the upper extreme of this specific cohort of patients and those at highest risk of complications.

The case series by Mannava et al. [18] included a cohort of 21 patients who participated in "fitness / weightlifting" activities prior to surgery. The average age across their cohort was 64 years old with a mean follow-up of 3.7 years. Results from the weightlifting cohort at final follow-up were 72.7% reporting an activity level "comparable with preoperative level of activity", 18.2% reporting an activity level "below preoperative level of activity" and 9.1% reporting they were "unable to participate". The case series conducted by Wang et al. [26] reported 19 of 27 (70%) patients were able to return to sport following aTSA, of which 7 patients returned to weight lifting. Six of the 7 patients reported they were active 1–3 times per week while the remaining patient was active in weightlifting 4–7 times per week. Unclear from this case series is how many weightlifting patients specifically were unable to return to sport following aTSA, and what degree of weightlifting was occurring.

The most elucidating evidence on weightlifting comes from a cohort study by Ames et al. [11] investigating the incidence of return to sport, patient reported outcomes, patient satisfaction, performance, and failures in a specific population of high demand weightlifters that continue lifting after undergoing total shoulder arthroplasty. Patients were advised not to continue heavy lifting following aTSA, however elected to proceed against surgeon advice. Heavy lifting was defined as preoperative bench pressing ≥200 lbs. (males) or ≥ 135 pounds (females); shoulder press ≥200 lbs. (males); competing professionally in sanctioned events; and/or lifting >3 days per week pre-operatively. Average age was 57.9 years and follow-up ranged from 1 to 7 years (average 3.6 years). Of the 42 shoulders included in the study, 23 of 36 patients (63.9%) reported a return to weightlifting 75-minutes per workout four times per week. The authors noted several important findings. First, there were zero patients required revision surgery. Second, there was an overall lower return to sport than previous case series reports of >70%. Third, the majority weightlifters were approaching 50% of pre-symptomatic bench press maximum and > 90% of pre-symptomatic latissimus pulldown maximum. Despite encouraging findings, the authors do not recommend surgeons change the current practice of recommending restrictions on weightlifting until further research is available. This would include mid-term or long-term outcomes in this high-demand patient population or further data on how weightlifting affects forces transmitted across implant interfaces. Lastly, the authors caution surgeons to anticipate that highly active, high-demand patients will likely attempt to return to sport against recommendations otherwise and may require additional counseling after TSA.

2.7 Anatomic total shoulder arthroplasty versus hemiarthroplasty

When treating glenohumeral arthritis, both hemiarthroplasty and total shoulder arthroplasty (**Figure 4**) have shown to be effective at managing pain and returning to sport. Historically, hemiarthroplasty has been viewed as the preferred treatment for younger, higher demand patients. Multiple survey studies have shown high levels of confidence in both HA and TSA when allowing return to sport, with >75% of respondents allowing return to sport for both patients, although respondents appeared more confident with return to sport in the HA (87.2% vs. 76.5%) [5].

While surgeons may have more confidence allowing return to sport following HA, literature appears to support that patients return to sport at a higher rate and more functional with TSA versus HA. A literature review performed by Christensen et al. [1] found a greater overall return to sport for TSA (57–96%) over HA (66–81%). An additional literature review by Johnson et al. [2] found similarly higher rates of return to sport following TSA (75–100%) over HA (67–76%). This has been confirmed in retrospective cohort studies. Garcia et al. [25] reviewed return to sport in a matched

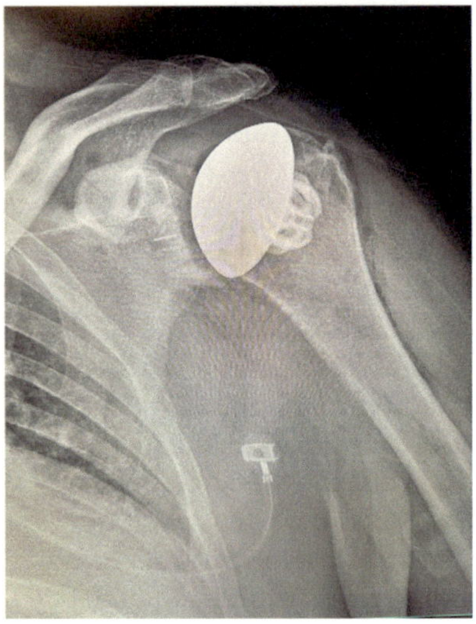

Figure 4.
Anatomic total shoulder arthroplasty.

cohort of patients who underwent TSA and HA and found significantly increased rates of return to sport in the TSA group (97.3% vs. 65.5%, $p < .001$), and return to higher upper extremity sports ($P = 0.01$). Wang et al. [26] also noted a higher rate of return to sport with TSA over HA (95% vs. 76%), the exception being in weightlifting where a higher percentage of HA patients were seen (59% vs. 37%), however no statistical analysis of significance was conducted. Other case series comparing the two groups have found no difference in return to sport [10, 12].

Patient satisfaction and patient reported outcomes tend to favor total shoulder arthroplasty over hemiarthroplasty in patients being treated for glenohumeral arthritis with no rotator cuff tears. The same conclusions should not be extrapolated to other indications for surgery. For example, a case control study comparing HA vs. TSA noted the statistically significant improvements in flexion, abduction and internal rotation, however the difference did not persist once patients who underwent hemiarthroplasty for indications such as rotator cuff tear, neoplasia, osteonecrosis and rotator cuff arthropathy were removed from the analysis [12]. The matched cohort study of patients with glenohumeral osteoarthritis found significant improvements in satisfaction with surgery (100% vs. 70%, $p = .01$) and satisfaction with sport (94.5% vs. 58.6%, $P < .001$) with TSA vs. HA [25]. The case series of patients being treated for osteoarthritis noted significant improvements in ASES in TSA patients, but no difference in SANE scores [26]. A large retrospective cohort conducted in the United Kingdom [27] reviewed patient reported outcomes using the Oxford Shoulder Score (OSS) in patients who underwent HA or TSA for osteoarthritis with intact cuffs. While both groups experienced a statistically significant from pre-op scores to 6-months, there was a statistically significant improvement in OSS favoring TSA over HA at 6-months. At 5-years, the mean OSS for TSA was 39.6 versus 32.6 for HA out of a possible score of 48. A more favorable OSS for TSA was also noted in patients under the age of 60 at 6 months post-op (TSA 37.1 +/− 9.8, HA 31.9 +/− 11.7). Lastly, a large meta-analysis of patients undergoing HA vs. TSA for glenohumeral osteoarthritis with intact rotator cuffs demonstrated a significant mean improvement in patient-reported outcomes in TSA over HA [15]. They also found a 2-fold increase in revision surgeries required for patients who underwent hemiarthroplasty (relative risk = 2.09, p = .01). This is consistent with prior studies investigating the longevity between HA and aTSA [1, 28]. They conclude TSA is favored over HA in terms of clinical outcome, risk of revision surgery and complications.

When selecting the operation best suited for a patient with glenohumeral arthritis and an intact rotator cuff, total shoulder arthroplasty appears to be the superior option over hemiarthroplasty. TSA shows increased return to sport rates and patients satisfaction. The optimal choice remains a patient-specific decision that depends on multiple factors including patients' age and activity demands, presence of glenoid arthritis as well as surgeon preference in their desire to preserve the glenoid or confidence with either procedure. HA and TSA can both provide patients with pain relief and return to certain sports at excellent rates. Both procedures come with their own drawbacks: HA can produce glenoid erosion and does not address glenoid-sided arthritis which may lead to incomplete resolution of symptoms while TSA may lead to glenoid component loosening and less bone stock for revision procedures if necessary. With improvements in glenoid technology and low rates of loosening data, newer data suggests that TSA may actually be appropriate for the younger, higher demand patient. Surgeon's should always caution patients about these risks of either procedure and patients involved in high-demand activities such as heavy weightlifting should understand that a return to pre-symptomatic level of participation may not be feasible, but advise that symptom relief and return to sport is likely following shoulder replacement.

2.8 Anatomic versus reverse total shoulder arthroplasty

Deciding between anatomic and reverse total shoulder arthroplasty generally boils down to the status of the patient's rotator cuff. RTSA was previously viewed as a salvage operation to assist with pain and overhead function in lower demand patients. Today, rTSA is gaining popularity and is the treatment of choice for patients with glenohumeral osteoarthritis and irreparable rotator cuff tears. Hemiarthroplasty may also be considered for patients with osteoarthritis and an irreparable rotator cuff. A non-functional rotator cuff is a contraindication to anatomic total shoulder arthroplasty as it leads to altered glenohumeral biomechanics, eccentric wear of the glenoid component. Patients undergoing rTSA are typically older than patients undergoing HA or aTSA and presumably have different activity level demands which may influence their rates of return to sport. Ultimately, rTSA is biomechanically different from HA or aTSA. It is semiconstrained and experiences unique forces at the joint as well as prosthesis-bone interface. Return to sport theoretically raises concerns about loss of fixation, accelerated wear, instability, deltoid fatigue, and acromial stress fractures.

Although consensus does not exist on protocols or which sports are acceptable following reverse total shoulder arthroplasty, overall this has been viewed cautiously by surgeons. In the survey conducted by Golant et al. [5], return to all sports was allowed by only 45.2% of respondents, compared with 76.5% and 87.2% for ATSA vs. HA respectively. Return to low-load sports (golfing, cycling, swimming, yoga) following rTSA was allowed by 72.2% of surgeons, whereas high-load (racket sports, softball/baseball, weightlifting, rock climbing and volleyball) were only allowed by 36.1% of respondents. This may reflect the lack of long term experience with rTSA as well as perceived high rate of complication.

This sentiment has been challenged by recent literature. Return to sport rates following rTSA have been reported to be between 60 and 86% [1]. A meta-analysis [8] comparing return to sport rates following aTSA vs. rTSA found a significantly lower return to sport rate for rTSA (77% vs. 90%, $p < 0.01$). A retrospective cohort study by Liu et al. [4] compared return to sport rates for patients with osteoarthritis and concomitant rotator cuff dysfunction who underwent either HA or rTSA. They found higher overall rates of return to sport in rTSA patients (85.9% vs. 66.7%, $P = 0.154$). They also found a significantly improved rate of return for rTSA versus HA for age < 70 years (96.8% vs. 65.0%) and when surgery was performed on the dominant extremity. A case series by Simovitch et al. [29] examined return to sport following rTSA in elderly patients with mean age 73+/− 7.2 years old and mean follow-up of 43+/− 12 months. They concluded a return to sport rate of 60% (40 of 67 patients). All patients had significant improvement in patient reported outcomes and range of motion. Seventy-three percent reported participating in more than one sport. Twelve patients (30%) performed at a higher level while 65% performed at the same level. They noted a 7% complication rate and 5% reoperation rate (1 P. Acnes infection and 1 dislocation while using the toilet). There were no patients who had component loosening and there were no unique failure modes identified. They concluded rTSA in senior athletes lead to significant clinical improvement without failure in short-term follow-up but recommended long-term studies with sport-specific stratification. A case series of patients who wished to return to racket sports prior to undergoing TSA or rTSA found an 80% return to sport rate in the rTSA group with no differences in amount played, range of motion, forehand, backhand or serving abilities when compared to aTSA [14]. Although promising, the rTSA cohort only included 13 patients. While aTSA appears to have the best rates of return to sport, reverse total shoulder arthroplasty is an acceptable option for elderly patients who wish to return to low-demand activities.

3. Complications following anatomic total shoulder arthroplasty

Complications following anatomic total shoulder arthroplasty include rotator cuff tears, subscapularis failure, aseptic glenoid or humeral component loosening, infection, instability, fracture or prolonged pain. Glenoid loosening is one of the most cited reasons for failure of aTSA. Fear of glenoid component failure drives the recommendation to restrict high demand activities in TSA patients. A large retrospective cohort study published in 2020 of 2224 aTSAs performed in the US and Europe utilizing a single implant identified 239 adverse events (10.7%) and 124 revisions (5.6%) [17]. The most common complication identified was subscapularis failure/rotator cuff tear (69 patients, 3.1% rate of all aTSA), resulting in 42 revision surgeries (1.9% of total cohort, 33.9% of all revisions). Glenoid loosening was identified in 55 patients (2.5% of total cohort) of which 42 required revision making it the most common cause of revision surgery (1.9% of cohort, 34.7% of revisions). The mean time to identification of glenoid loosening was 55.8 +/− 45.1 months. This study was strictly investigating numbers and rates of complication and did not mention activity level or participation in sports.

While glenoid loosening is the most common cause of revision surgery, multiple case series with short to medium term follow-up do not support this claim. Ames et al. [11] demonstrated no patients requiring revision TSA and no evidence of glenoid loosening at 3.6 year follow-up in a high-demand cohort of athletes. In a study by Garcia et al. [3] evaluating RTS in patients <55 years old undergoing TSA, there were high rates of return to fitness and high demand sports and at average 61-month

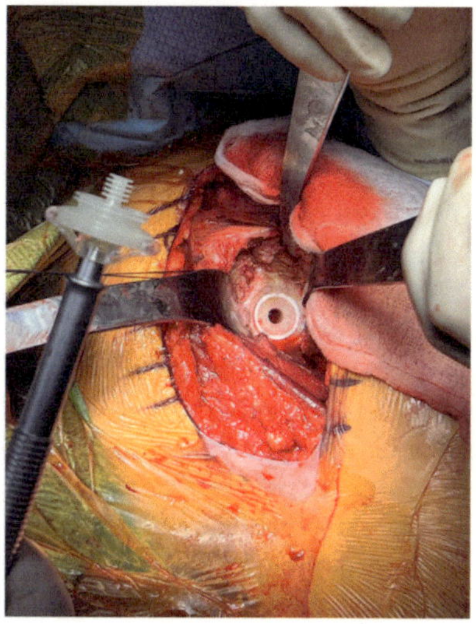

Figure 5.
Intraoperative view of glenoid exposure.

follow-up no patients required glenoid component revision. Another study by Shimada et al. [30] evaluated 90 shoulders (60 underwent rTSA). This study found only one developed glenoid component loosening at midterm follow up despite high return to sport rate. A case series by Yalcin et al. [13] on 16 elite weightlifters, 17 shoulders, treated for osteoarthritis using a novel aTSA implant consisting of a nonspherical humeral head and inlay glenoid replacement showed zero revision surgeries at 38 months f/u. Fifteen of sixteen patients returned to same or heavy weightlifting post-operatively (94%).

Attention to the patient's anatomy, a thorough review or preoperative imaging, meticulous planning and proper intra-operative technique allowing proper glenoid exposure (**Figure 5**) is paramount, especially in higher demand athletes. Surgeons should avoid over medialization and excessive retroversion. Implants should obtain near full backside support and if positioned in too much retroversion or superior inclination risk edge loading [31]. Newer glenoid designs, such as posterior augments, peg design or inlay/inset, should be familiar to the surgeon and utilized when appropriate. Future studies are required prior to making recommendations on the superiority of one design in terms of glenoid loosening.

Without long term radiographic follow-up, the authors do not recommend changing practice. While caution is still advised with returning to higher demand activities like heavy weightlifting, the current data highlights the positives of modern fixation techniques. Long-term studies evaluating the durability and survivorship of TSA in younger patients and high demand athletes should be conducted. Further studies may help surgeons educate patients and allow discussion regarding return to sport after shoulder arthroplasty.

4. Conclusions

Anatomic total shoulder arthroplasty (aTSA) is becoming an increasingly common method of treating glenohumeral arthritis in younger patients with intact rotator cuffs. The patient population undergoing aTSA has evolved into people who are not just hopeful for pain control, but to return to an active lifestyle. Return to sport rates in lower demand sports in recent literature has been very promising, with rates ranging from 75 to 100% being reported [1–4]. Return to sport rates and patient satisfaction appear to favor aTSA over hemiarthroplasty (HA), however HA is appropriate under certain indications. Increased rates of return to higher demand sports such as tennis and weightlifting have also been seen in newer literature, however surgeons agreed that these activities should be approached cautiously and on a case-by-case basis. A consensus on recovery protocol following surgery does not currently exist, but the literature generally supports a few key points: (1) Extremes of passive external rotation should be avoided early on; (2) return to sport should only be considered once a patient has met their goals for range of motion, strength, and painlessly execution of sport-specific activities; and (3) return to sport should be avoided until 3 months after surgery. While revision rates for aTSA remain relatively low (5.6%) [17] and glenoid loosening rates may be declining due to improved surgical techniques and improved technology, patients who wish to undergo total shoulder arthroplasty should be counseled thoroughly on them prior to surgery. Further investigation into return to high-demand sports and glenoid component loosening in athletic populations following total shoulder arthroplasty is necessary to strengthen these findings.

Author details

Neal Krentz[1], Benjamin Sanderford[1], Kelly Wolfe[1] and Andrew Ames[2]*

1 McLaren Oakland, Pontiac, Michigan, United States of America

2 Orthopedic Specialists of Oakland County, Bloomfield Hills, Michigan, United States of America

*Address all correspondence to: aames@osoc.com

References

[1] Christensen J, Brockmeier S. Total shoulder arthroplasty in the athlete and active individual. Clinics in Sports Medicine. 2018;**37**(4):549-558

[2] Johnson CC, Johnson DJ, Liu JN, Dines JS, Dines DM, Gulotta LV, et al. Return to sports after shoulder arthroplasty. World Journal of Orthopedics. 2016;7(9):519-526

[3] Garcia GH, Liu JN, Sinatro A, Wu HH, Dines JS, Warren RF, et al. High satisfaction and return to sports after total shoulder arthroplasty in patients aged 55 years and younger. The American Journal of Sports Medicine. 2017;**45**(7):1664-1669

[4] Liu JN, Steinhaus ME, Garcia GH, Chang B, Fields K, Dines DM, et al. Return to sport after shoulder arthroplasty: A systematic review and meta-analysis. Knee Surgery, Sports Traumatology, Arthroscopy. 2018;**26**(1):100-112

[5] Golant A, Christoforou D, Zuckerman JD, Kwon YW. Return to sports after shoulder arthroplasty: A survey of surgeons' preferences. Journal of Shoulder and Elbow Surgery. 2012;**21**(4):554-560

[6] Healy WL, Iorio R, Lemos MJ. Athletic activity after joint replacement. The American Journal of Sports Medicine. 2001;**29**(3):377-388

[7] Magnussen RA, Mallon WJ, Willems WJ, Moorman CT. Long-term activity restrictions after shoulder arthroplasty: An international survey of experienced shoulder surgeons. Journal of Shoulder and Elbow Surgery. 2011;**20**(2):281-289

[8] Papalia R, Ciuffreda M, Albo E, De Andreis C, Diaz Balzani LA, Alifano AM, et al. Return to sport after anatomic and reverse total shoulder arthroplasty in elderly patients: A systematic review and meta-analysis. Journal of Clinical Medicine. 2020;**9**(5):1576

[9] Farley KX, Wilson JM, Kumar A, Gottschalk MB, Daly C, Sanchez-Sotelo J, et al. Prevalence of shoulder arthroplasty in the United States and the increasing burden of revision shoulder arthroplasty. JBJS Open Access. 2021;**6**(3):e20.00156

[10] McCarty EC, Marx RG, Maerz D, Altchek D, Warren RF. Sports participation after shoulder replacement surgery. The American Journal of Sports Medicine. 2008;**36**(8):1577-1581

[11] Ames A, Shah S, Pettit R, Li L, Chilton M, Alnusif N, et al. Against surgeons' advice: The return to sport in high demand weightlifters following anatomic total shoulder arthroplasty at average 3.6 years follow-up. Journal of Shoulder and Elbow Surgery. 2023;**32**(4):153-159

[12] Zarkadas PC, Throckmorton TQ, Dahm DL, Sperling J, Schleck CD, Cofield R. Patient reported activities after shoulder replacement: Total and hemiarthroplasty. Journal of Shoulder and Elbow Surgery. 2011;**20**(2):273-280

[13] Yalcin S, Scarcella M, Everhart J, Samuel L, Miniaci A. Clinical and radiographic outcomes of Total shoulder arthroplasty with a nonspherical humeral head and inlay glenoid in elite weight lifters: A prospective case series. Orthopaedic Journal of Sports Medicine. 2021;**9**(7):23259671211021055

[14] Vegas A, Cannon D, Rafael Garcia J, Rodriguez HC, Levy J, Lapica H, et al. Return to racket sports after shoulder arthroplasty: Performance and outcome scores. Seminars in Arthroplasty: JSES. 2023;**33**(3):447-454

[15] Singh Jagdev B, McGrath J, Cole A, Gomaa AR, Chong HH, Singh HP. Total shoulder arthroplasty vs. hemiarthroplasty in patients with primary glenohumeral arthritis with intact rotator cuff: Meta-analysis using the ratio of means. Journal of Shoulder and Elbow Surgery. 2022;**31**(12):2657-2670

[16] Bhat SB, Lazarus M, Getz C, Williams GR, Namdari S. Economic decision model suggests total shoulder arthroplasty is superior to hemiarthroplasty in young patients with end-stage shoulder arthritis. Clinical Orthopaedics. 2016;**474**(11):2482-2492

[17] Parada SA, Flurin PH, Wright TW, Zuckerman JD, Elwell JA, Roche CP, et al. Comparison of complication types and rates associated with anatomic and reverse total shoulder arthroplasty. Journal of Shoulder and Elbow Surgery. 2021;**30**(4):811-818

[18] Mannava S, Horan MP, Frangiamore SJ, Hussain ZB, Fritz EM, Godin JA, et al. Return to recreational sporting activities following total shoulder arthroplasty. Orthopaedic Journal of Sports Medicine. 2018;**6**(7):2325967118782672

[19] Bülhoff M, Sattler P, Bruckner T, Loew M, Zeifang F, Raiss P. Do patients return to sports and work after total shoulder replacement surgery? The American Journal of Sports Medicine. 2015;**43**(2):423-427

[20] Mehta N, Acuna AJ, McCormick JR, Harkin WE, Swindell HW, Defroda SF, et al. Publicly available anatomic total shoulder arthroplasty rehabilitation protocols show high variability and frequent divergence from the 2020 ASSET recommendations. International Journal of Sports Physical Therapy. 2024;**19**(7):856-867

[21] Bornes TD, Rollins MD, Lapner PL, Bouliane MJ. Subscapularis management in total shoulder arthroplasty: Current evidence comparing peel, osteotomy, and tenotomy. Journal of Shoulder and Elbow Arthroplasty. 2018;**2**:2471549218807772

[22] Kennedy JS, Garrigues GE, Pozzi F, Zens MJ, Gaunt B, Phillips B, et al. The American society of shoulder and elbow therapists' consensus statement on rehabilitation for anatomic total shoulder arthroplasty. Journal of Shoulder and Elbow Surgery. 2020;**29**(10):2149-2162

[23] Jensen KL, Rockwood CA. Shoulder arthroplasty in recreational golfers. Journal of Shoulder and Elbow Surgery. 1998;**7**(4):362-367

[24] Schumann K, Flury MP, Schwyzer HK, Simmen BR, Drerup S, Goldhahn J. Sports activity after anatomical total shoulder arthroplasty. The American Journal of Sports Medicine. 2010;**38**(10):2097-2105

[25] Garcia GH, Liu JN, Mahony GT, Sinatro A, Wu HH, Craig EV, et al. Hemiarthroplasty versus total shoulder arthroplasty for shoulder osteoarthritis: A matched comparison of return to sports. The American Journal of Sports Medicine. 2016;**44**(6):1417-1422

[26] Wang J, Popchak A, Giugale J, Irrgang J, Lin A. Sports participation is an appropriate expectation for recreational athletes undergoing shoulder arthroplasty. Orthopaedic Journal of Sports Medicine. 2018;**6**(10):2325967118800666

[27] Davies AR, Sabharwal S, Liddle AD, Zamora-Talaya B, Rangan A, Reilly P. Patient-reported outcomes following total shoulder arthroplasty and hemiarthroplasty: An analysis of data from the national joint registry. Journal of Shoulder and Elbow Surgery. 2024;**33**(11):2411-2420

[28] Sperling JW, Cofield RH, Rowland CM. Minimum fifteen-year follow-up of neer hemiarthroplasty and total shoulder arthroplasty in patients aged fifty years or younger. Journal of Shoulder and Elbow Surgery. 2004;**13**(6):604-613

[29] Simovitch RW, Gerard BK, Brees JA, Fullick R, Kearse JC. Outcomes of reverse total shoulder arthroplasty in a senior athletic population. Journal of Shoulder and Elbow Surgery. 2015;**24**(9):1481-1485

[30] Shimada Y, Matsuki K, Sugaya H, Takahashi N, Tokai M, Hashimoto E, et al. Return to sports and physical work after anatomical and reverse shoulder arthroplasty. Journal of Shoulder and Elbow Surgery. 2023;**32**(7):1445-1451

[31] Wright MA, O'Leary M, Johnston P, Murthi AM. Advances in anatomic total shoulder arthroplasty glenoid implant design. The Journal of the American Academy of Orthopaedic Surgeons. 2025;**33**(2):56-64